FMGE/NEET PG REVIEW 2019

285 Latest Questions With Explanations of FMGE June 2019

FMGE/NEET PG REVIEW 2019

285 Latest Questions With Explanations of FMGE June 2019

Armaan Chourasiya (Bhupendra)
CEO
MCI Gurukul
New Delhi, India

JAYPEE

JAYPEE BROTHERS MEDICAL PUBLISHERS
The Health Sciences Publisher
New Delhi | London

Jaypee Brothers Medical Publishers (P) Ltd

Headquarters

Jaypee Brothers Medical Publishers (P) Ltd
4838/24, Ansari Road, Daryaganj
New Delhi 110 002, India
Phone: +91-11-43574357
Fax: +91-11-43574314
Email: jaypee@jaypeebrothers.com

Overseas Office

J.P. Medical Ltd
83 Victoria Street, London
SW1H 0HW (UK)
Phone: +44 20 3170 8910
Fax: +44 (0)20 3008 6180
Email: info@jpmedpub.com

Website: www.jaypeebrothers.com
Website: www.jaypeedigital.com

FMGE/NEET PG Review 2019

First edition: **2019**

ISBN 978-93-89587-90-6
Printed at Replika Press Pvt. Ltd.

Dedicated to

Almighty God
My parents,
My father OP Chourasiya and
My mother Indu Chourasiya
Brother Neeraj and Sister Deepika
and FMGE/NEET-PG/MBBS aspirants
of India and abroad

Preface

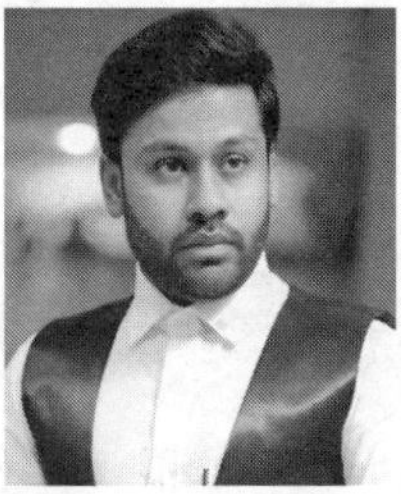

Before telling you about the book and the pattern of examination I will give you one genuine advice.

"Never do tomorrow what you can do today. Procrastination is the thief of time", and remember one more important thing.

"You may encounter many defeats, but you must not be defeated. In fact, it may be necessary to encounter the defeats, so you can know who you are, what you can rise from, how you can still come out of it."

NBE questions are most challenging, most important and believe me, the most nerve wrecking now a days.

Question of NBE as most of us know, are never straight forward, never directly factual but are utterly conceptual. It requires through knowledge of the basics of the subjects.

By detailed analysis and experience of most, it has been proved without any doubt that NBE Question bank which is the base of clearing FMGE (Foreign Medical Graduate Examination/ NEET PG Entrance/DNB). NBE question bank is the most trendy, awake to recent changes in treatment profile, drug of choice, investigation of choice etc.

Questions of NBE are framed after thorough research, to test our knowledge of the subjects matter, how we exclude closely related condition and our intellect to choose the right answer based on the deep conceptual knowledge of various clinical condition, rather than meaningless mugging up the attributes of disease and characteristic of different topics.

This book basically telling you the latest framing of questions by NBE which will be helpful for all aspirants, because it will tell you the topics, content, and importantly the depth till NBE questions will penetrate.

Also remember, when I am talking about NBE Question bank it means I am talking about all three important examination conducted by National Board of Examination.

1. FMGE
2. NEET PG
3. DNB

Acknowledgments

First, thanks to my family for having the patience in me for taking yet another challenge which decreases the amount of time I can spend with them, especially my father (Er. OP Chourasiya) and mother (Mrs Indu Chourasiya) and my brothers Er Neeraj Chourasiya (Director MCI Gurukul Delhi and MBBS Gurukul Abroad Education and Services) Mentor, Motivator and Dr Vishal Chourasiya DM (Liver Transplant), MS, MBBS. Both of them are my biggest inspiration and motivation to improve my knowledge and move my career forward continuously. My Grandparents, who rests in peace, late Janki Prasad Chourasiya and late Shanti Devi Chourasiya, late Rampyari Bai Chourasiya and late Dharbhari Lal Ji Chourasiya.

Their blessings are always with me and motivating me for improving my attitude towards my profession and share credit on my success.

Special thanks to my uncle Mr Anoop Chourasiya and Er Rajesh Chourasiya, and aunty Mrs Pratibha Chourasiya, my cute younger brother Harsh Chourasiya (Bitta).

I would like to thank my elder brothers Dr Prashant Ranjan Mishra (ASMI, Vice Rector) and Dr Umesh Srivastava for standing beside me.

My brother Er Rahul Chourasiya, Director (MBBS Gurukul Central India), my bosom friend and brother Mr Sohaib Khan, my brother Mr Suneel Verma, my elder brother Mr Rajesh Mishra and all MCI Gurukul and MBBS Gurukul staff all over the world.

I would like to acknowledge the MCI Gurukul Legendary Faculty Team of India.

Alllegends under one roof in “MCI Gurukul Delhi”

1. Dr Gobind Rai Garg (Pharmacology)
2. Dr Vivek Jain (PSM)
3. Dr Deepak Marwah (Medicine)
4. Dr Sakshi Arora (OBG)
5. Dr Sparsh Gupta (Pathology)
6. Dr Apurv Mehra (Orthopedic)
7. Dr Soumen Manna/Dr Krishna Kumar (Physiology)
8. Dr Akhilesh Raj Jhamad (FMT and Dermatology)
9. Dr Sonu Panwar (Microbiology)

10. Dr Dharmendra/Dr Nilesh Chandra (Biochemistry)
11. Dr Pritesh Singh/Dr Nachiketa (Surgery)
12. Dr Sarvejeet Singh/Dr Sanjay Agarwal (ENT)
13. Dr Zainab Bora (Radiology)
14. Dr Rajesh Kaushal/Dr Arnika Singhal/Dr Raviraj (Anatomy)
15. Dr Utsav Bansal/Dr Rajarathna (Ophthalmology)
16. Dr Singaram Ashok (Pediatric)
17. Dr Dharmendra/Dr Praveen (Psychiatry)
18. Dr Ashish Ranjan (Anesthesia)

I would like to extend my warm regards to my cousins and friends

Dr Saurabh Tiwari (Fortis)
Dr Rakesh (ENT)
Dr Vinay (Author DNB)
Dr Akhilesh
Dr Arun
Dr Anil (NIE)
Dr Umesh Patel (BMC)
Dr Anjali Virani (BMC)
Mr Anush
Ms Ritu
Mr Vineet (Vini)
Mr Bhupesh S
Mr Satendra
Mr Shailesh
Mr Sandeep
Dr Manu
Mr Somesh
Mr Mahesh
Mr Vishal (Ashok Nagar)
Er Navin
Er Nitin
Mr Rahul
Mr Kuldeep
Er Pramod
Er Vikas
Mr Rajeev
Mr Manish
Mr Pankaj
Mr Sameer
Mrs Sonika
Mrs Shanu
Mrs Mamta
Ms Megha
Mrs Deepa
Mrs Rani
Ms Namrata (Puna)
Dr Ankit Jain
Dr Shivalik Gupta
Dr Manthan Purohit
Dr Baljeet Singh
Dr Sanam
Dr Chirag Pujara
Dr Eliyas
Dr Nasmal
Dr Richa
Dr Nitin

I feel immense pleasure in conveying my sincere thanks to my relatives.

Dr Vinod–Mrs Sakuntalla (Neemuch)

Mr Kailash–Mrs Geeta (Ashok Nagar)

Mr Anoop–Mrs Sushma (Neemuch)

Er Rajesh–Mrs Pratibha (Bhopal)

Mr Jeevan–Mrs Pramila (Indore)
Dr Vedprakash–Mrs Uma (Meerut)
Dr Vishal–Dr Pratibha (Delhi)
Dr Varsha–Mr Rahul (Delhi)
Dr Kaku–Dr Nadia (Bhopal)
Mr Purushotam–Mrs Rekha (Bhopal)
Dr Dharmendra (Ortho)–Dr Satish Raghuwanshi
Mr Raj–Mrs Rakhi (Gwalior)
Dr Neema–Dr Surendra Pal (Meerut)
Mr Jeetendra–Mr Sanjeev (Ajmer)

I would like to thank Shri Jitendar P Vij (Group Chairman), Mr Ankit Vij (Managing Director), Ms Chetna Malhotra Vohra (Associate Director-Content Strategy), Ms Payal Bharti (Sr Manager, Publishing), Ms Ruby Sharma (Project Manager), Mr Himanshu (Proof Reader), Mr Rajesh Saini (DTP Operator) and the staff of M/s Jaypee Brothers Medical Publishers (P) Ltd, New Delhi, India, for their whole hearted support and encouragement in publishing the book.

I also extend my sincere thanks to all respective members of particular colleges I am mentioning.

Dr Umesh Srivastava and Dr Prashant Ranjan Mishra (Vice-Rector) of Asian Medical Institute, Kant, Kyrgyzstan)
Dr Bhupendra Kumar Magarde
Dr Waseem Khan Changwani, (Osh State University)
Dr Washim Sayed (Tver) and Dr Juwell (Osh State University, Kyrgyzstan)
Dr Shoaib Shahid (Vice Dean JSMU)
Dr Pradeep (Jalalabad State Medical University, Kyrgyzstan)
Dr Mehraj (Bashkir State Medical University)
Dr Alok Aeron (Smolensk State Medical University)
Dr Dharmendra (Ulyanovsk State Medical University)
Mr Niraj Nishchal (Mordovia State University)
Mr Ashutosh (Kazaan State Medical University)
Dr Kuldeep Sharma, Kursk State Medical University, Russia
Dr Amreek Singh Dhillon (Uzhhorod National Medical University, Ukraine) and Mr Harmeek Singh Dhillon
Dr Sudhir Dhakre and Dr Ashu Rawat (Odessa National Medical University, Ukraine)

Mr Hardeep Singh and Mr Sachin Kaushik (VN Karazina Kharkov National Medical University)

Mr Afzal (Sumy State University)

Mr Sumit Lamba and Mr Puneet Kumar (Ternopil National Medical University)

Dr Navdeep Singh and Dr Anil Dayal (Vinnysta State Medical University)

Dr Masroor Ahamad (Ivano Frankivsk National Medical University [IFNMU]

Mr Om Prakash (Ukraine Medical Stomatological Academy)

Dr Varun Malhotra (Zaporozhye State Medical University)

Mr Sandeep (OO Bogomolets)

Mr Alakh Singh (Dnipropetrovsk State Medical academy)

Dr Sunil Sharma (Bukovinian State Medical University)

Dr Junaid Malik (YSMU, Armenia)

Mr Vivek Jaiswal, Mr Sidharth Jaiswal (AMA)

Dr Jinghal Zhu, Dr Bochen Pan (Dean, China Medical University), Dr Fengrong and Mrs QuMin (CMU, Shenyang)

Dr Varshit Reddy and Er Harshit Reddy (Bright Education, Hyderabad)

Dr Muhammed Hassan, Dr Sreejith, Dr Lejoe Thomas (Dr SOS Pvt Ltd.)

Dr Om Sah, Dr Pradeep and Er Kavindra (Beihua University)

Dr Shaochun (Vice Dean, Kunming Medical University)

Mr N. Srinivasa Rao (Zhengzhou University)

Mr Pawan Kumar (Meta Education)

Dr TN Dubey (DM), Dr RN Sahu (Professor and HOD Psychiatry)

Dr Jay Prakash Agarwal (Assistant Professor)

Dr Radhvendra Singh Meena (Assistant Professor)

Dr BS Yadav (Professor Department of Cardiology)

Dr Sanjeev Kumar Shrivastava (Physiology)

Dr Ranjeet Singh Arya (Anatomy)

Dr Nitin Nahar (Assistant Professor) of Gandhi Medical College, Bhopal

Finally this book is a tribute to my best friend Late Ankit Dixit, may his soul rest in peace.

Who can study this book?

This book is must for all medical aspirants who are focusing to crack NBE conducted examination.

1. FMGE
2. NEET PG
3. DNB

All can study this latest 285 Questions with Explanations of FMGE June 2019.

NBE conducting all 3 examinations, so remember one thing of mine, If you are a NEET-PG aspirants and want to crack NEET-PG, you have to study recent questions of FMGE and DNB as well as with previous questions of NEET-PG.

Same with FMGE aspirants, who are studying for FMGE and want to crack FMGE, they have to study recent paper of NEET-PG, FMGE and DNB as well.

Anyone who is focusing DNB, has to study recent questions of FMGE and NEET-PG as well.

From this new pattern one thing is clear name of the examinations are different but the question pattern and image-based questions of all these 3 examinations are almost same.

Even if somebody is preparing for AIIMS-PG can have a look of this new pattern by NBE in which you will also get 60+ image-based questions which can come in AIIMS examination also.

As the pattern is same for all three examinations now a days, I am mentioning the blue prints of all subjects for FMGE Dec 2019 and NEET PG Jan 2020 together.

Study according to this preference of subjects as I am mentioning in the Blueprints.

Subjects	Questions asked in NEET PG	Questions asked in FMGE
1. Anatomy	15	17
2. Physiology	15	17
3. Biochemistry	15	17
4. Pathology	25	13
5. Pharmacology	20	13
6. Microbiology	20	13
7. Forensic medicine	10	10
8. ENT	10	15
9. PSM	25	30
10. Ophthalmology	10	15
11. Psychiatry	10	05
12. Orthopedics	15	05
13. Radiology	10	10
14. Dermatology	6-8	05
15. Anesthesia	6-8	05
16. Pediatrics	15	15
17. OBG	25	30
18. Medicine	30	33
19. Surgery	28	32

So all the best to
All of you facing coming
FMGE/AIIMS-PG/NEET-PG/DNB

References

References are taken from the latest edition of following books

Anatomy: Gray's Anatomy 41st edition

Physiology: Guyton and Hall 13th edition

Biochemistry: Harpers Illustrated Biochemistry 31st edition

Embryology: Langman's Medical Embryology 11th edition

Pathology: Robbins Basic Pathology 10th edition

Pharmacology: Essentials of Medical Pharmacology KDT 8th edition

Microbiology: Ananthanarayan and Paniker's Textbook of Microbiology 10th edition

Forensic: Review of Forensic Medicine and Toxicology 4th edition

PSM: Park's Textbook of Preventive and Social Medicine 25th edition

Ophthalmology: Comprehensive ophthalmology by AK khurana 7th edition

ENT: Dhingra's Diseases of ENT 7th edition

Orthopedics: Rockwood and Green's Fractures in Adults 8th edition

Anesthesia: Morgan and Mikhail's Clinical Anesthesiology, 6th edition

Radiology: The Basics and Fundamentals of Imaging 4th edition

Psychiatry: Diagnostic and Statistical Manual of Mental Disorders 5th edition

Dermatology: Clinical Dermatology 5th edition

Medicine: Harrison's Principles of Internal Medicine 20th edition

OBG: DC Dutta's Textbook of Obstetrics 9th edition

Surgery: Bailey and Love's Short Practice of Surgery 27th edition

Pediatrics: OP Ghai Pediatrics 10th edition

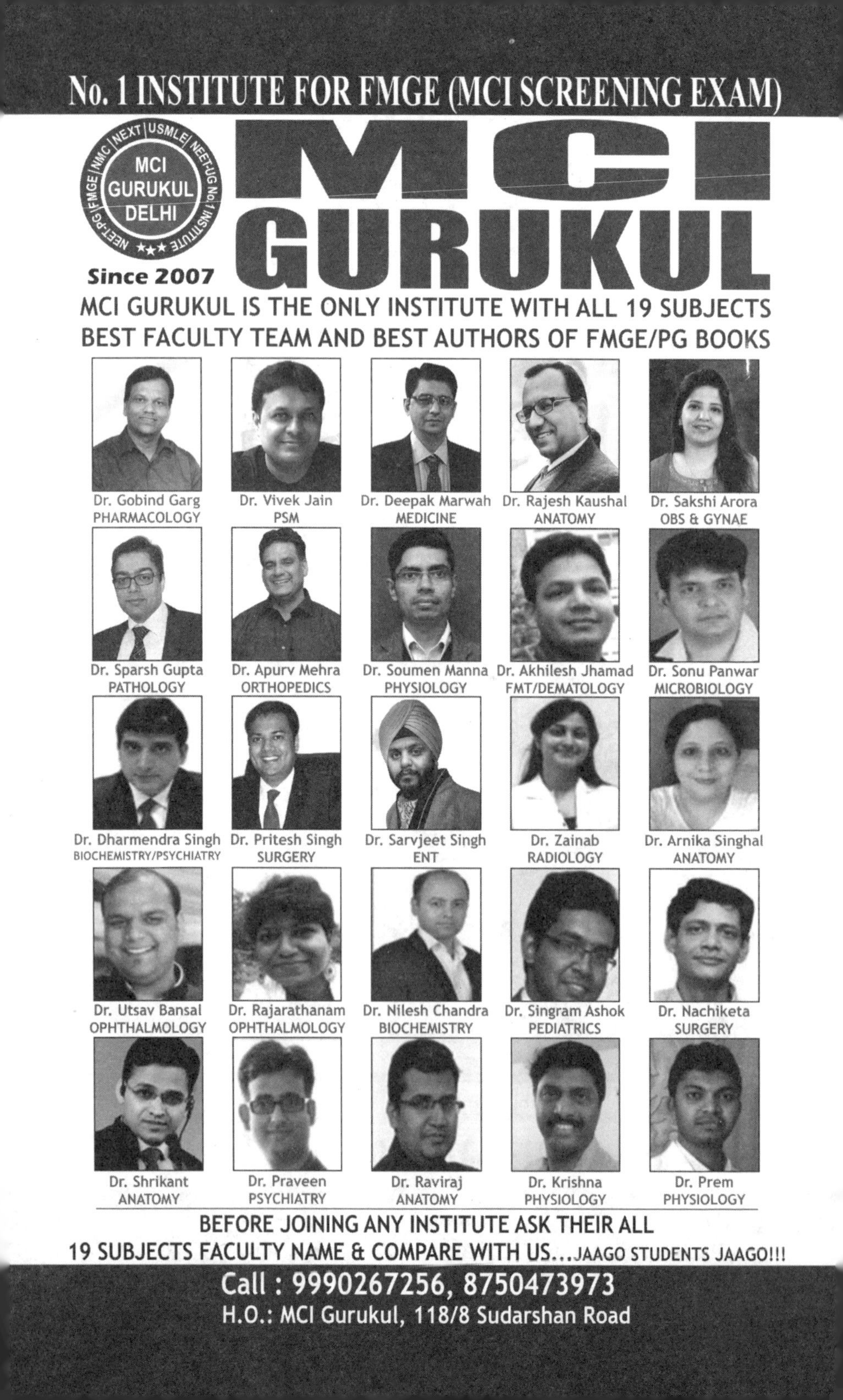
No. 1 INSTITUTE FOR FMGE (MCI SCREENING EXAM)
MCI GURUKUL DELHI
NEXT | USMLE | NEET-UG No.1 INSTITUTE | NEET-PG | FMGE | NMC
Since 2007
MCI GURUKUL
MCI GURUKUL IS THE ONLY INSTITUTE WITH ALL 19 SUBJECTS
BEST FACULTY TEAM AND BEST AUTHORS OF FMGE/PG BOOKS
Dr. Gobind Garg PHARMACOLOGY
Dr. Vivek Jain PSM
Dr. Deepak Marwah MEDICINE
Dr. Rajesh Kaushal ANATOMY
Dr. Sakshi Arora OBS & GYNAE
Dr. Sparsh Gupta PATHOLOGY
Dr. Apurv Mehra ORTHOPEDICS
Dr. Soumen Manna PHYSIOLOGY
Dr. Akhilesh Jhamad FMT/DEMATOLOGY
Dr. Sonu Panwar MICROBIOLOGY
Dr. Dharmendra Singh BIOCHEMISTRY/PSYCHIATRY
Dr. Pritesh Singh SURGERY
Dr. Sarvjeet Singh ENT
Dr. Zainab RADIOLOGY
Dr. Arnika Singhal ANATOMY
Dr. Utsav Bansal OPHTHALMOLOGY
Dr. Rajarathanam OPHTHALMOLOGY
Dr. Nilesh Chandra BIOCHEMISTRY
Dr. Singram Ashok PEDIATRICS
Dr. Nachiketa SURGERY
Dr. Shrikant ANATOMY
Dr. Praveen PSYCHIATRY
Dr. Raviraj ANATOMY
Dr. Krishna PHYSIOLOGY
Dr. Prem PHYSIOLOGY
BEFORE JOINING ANY INSTITUTE ASK THEIR ALL
19 SUBJECTS FACULTY NAME & COMPARE WITH US...JAAGO STUDENTS JAAGO!!!
Call : 9990267256, 8750473973
H.O.: MCI Gurukul, 118/8 Sudarshan Road

Contents

Color Plates (Image-based Questions)

MCQs with Explanations—June 2019 **1–106**

IMAGE-BASED QUESTIONS

Plate 1

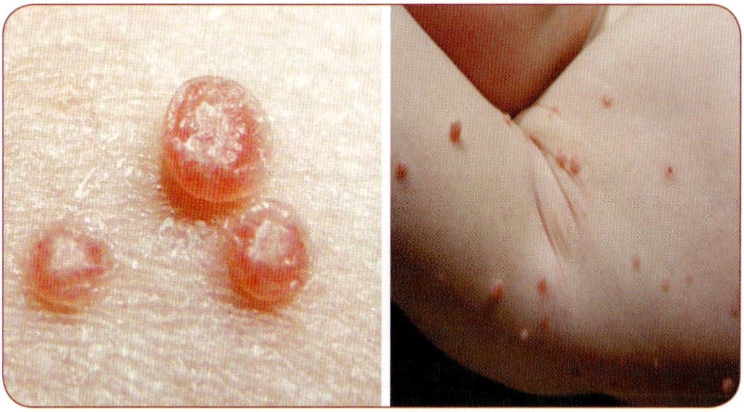

Question No. 262
Answer: Molluscum contagiosum

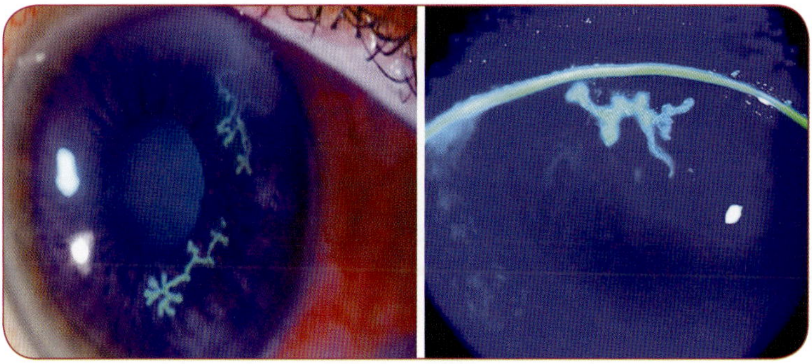

Question No. 263
Answer: Herpetic epithelial keratitis

Plate 2

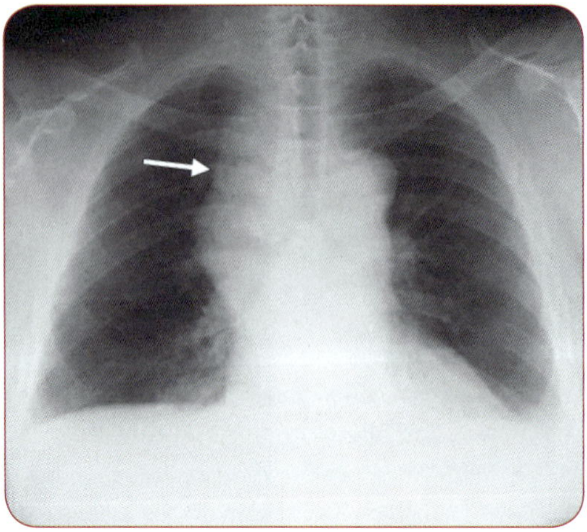

Question No. 264
Answer: Massive pleural effusion

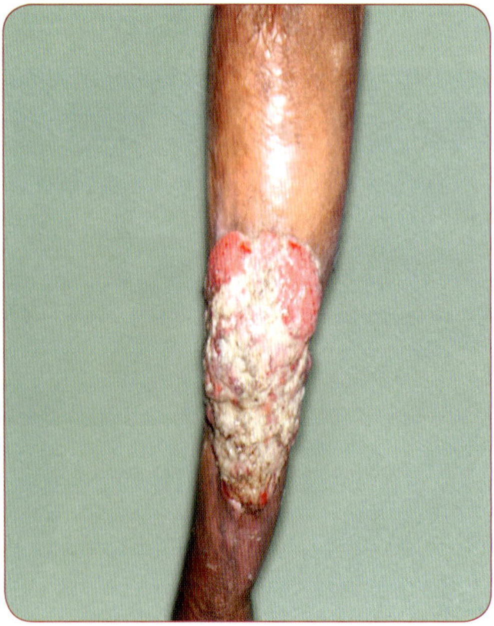

Question No. 265
Answer: Marjolin ulcer

Plate 3

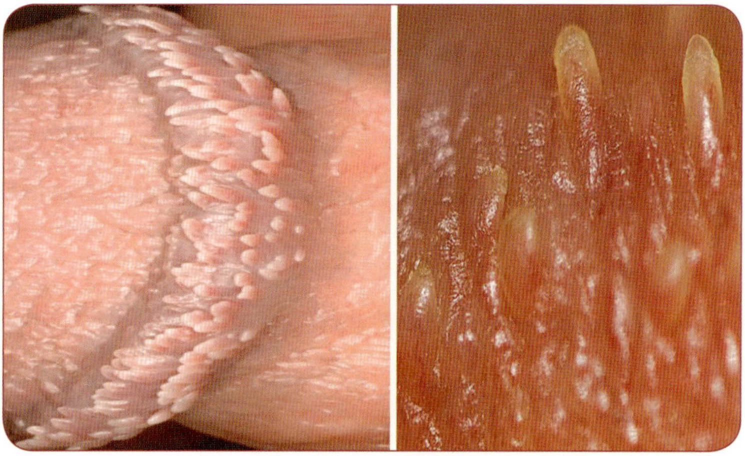

Question No. 266
Answer: Pearly penile papules

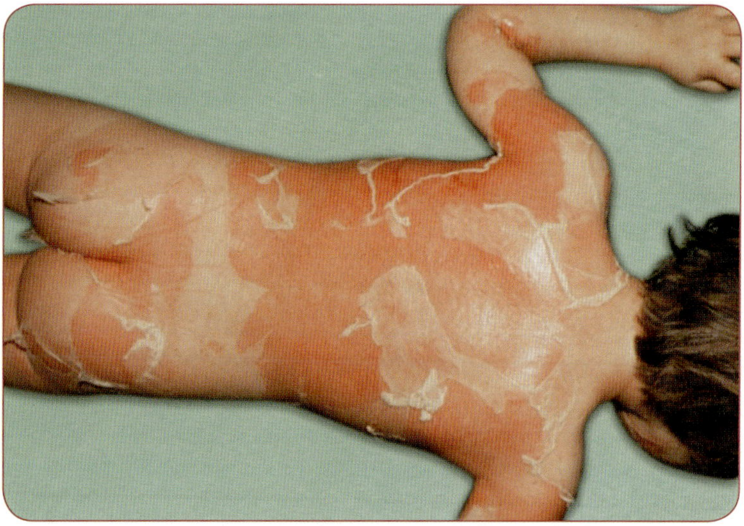

Question No. 267
Answer: Staphylococcal scalded skin syndrome

Plate 4

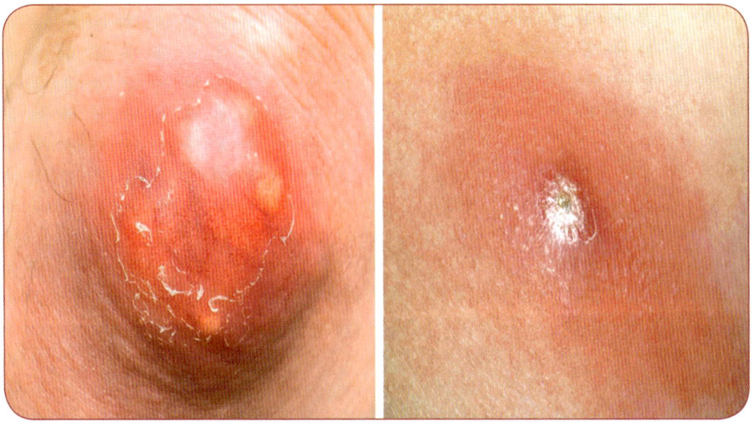

Question No. 268
Answer: Boils

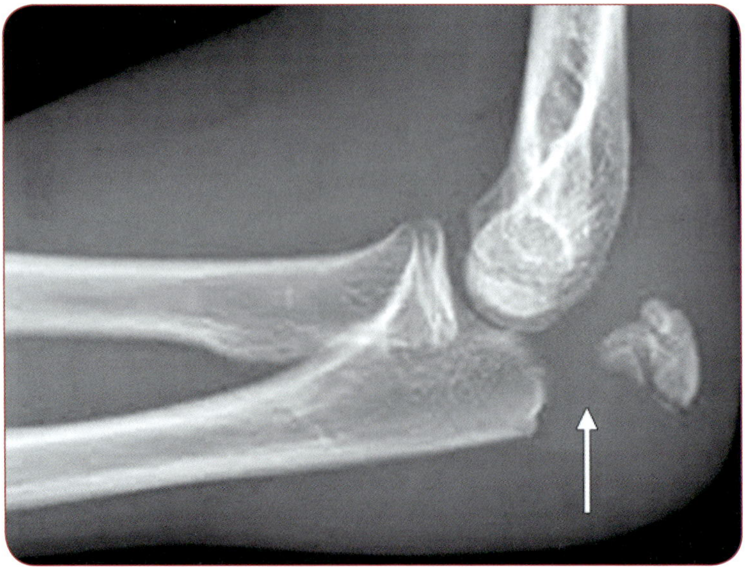

Question No. 269
Answer: Olecranon fracture

Plate 5

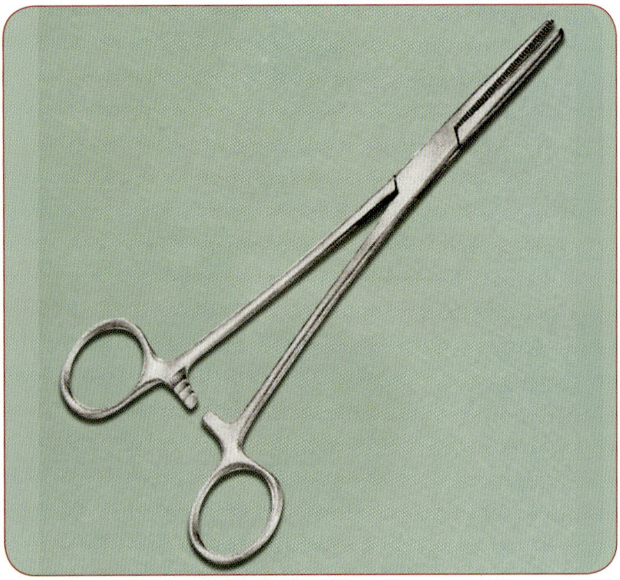

Question No. 270
Answer: Artery forcep

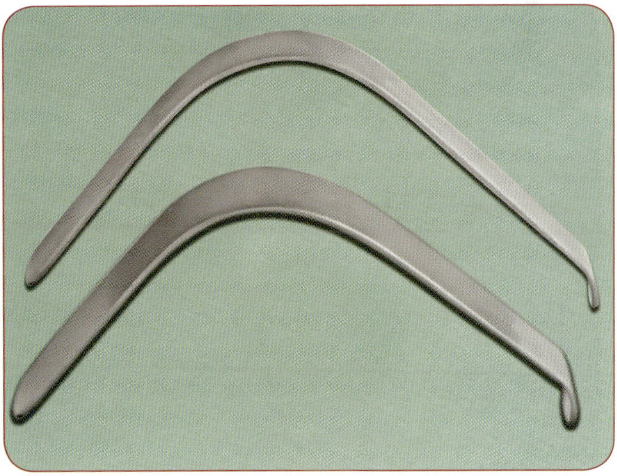

Question No. 271
Answer: Lack Tongue Depressor

Plate 6

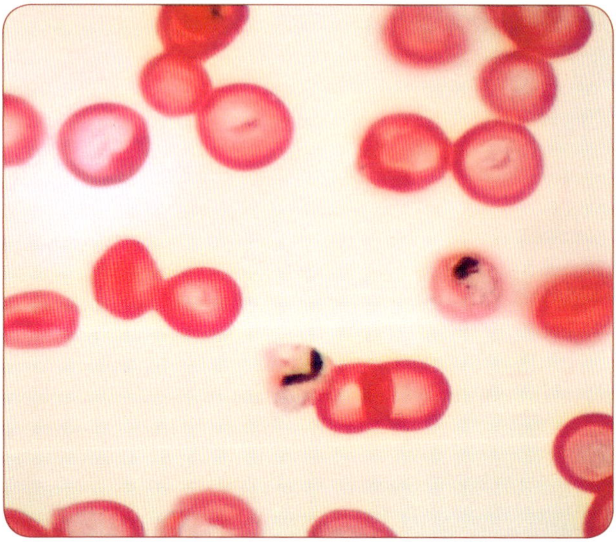

Question No. 272
Answer: *P. falciparum*

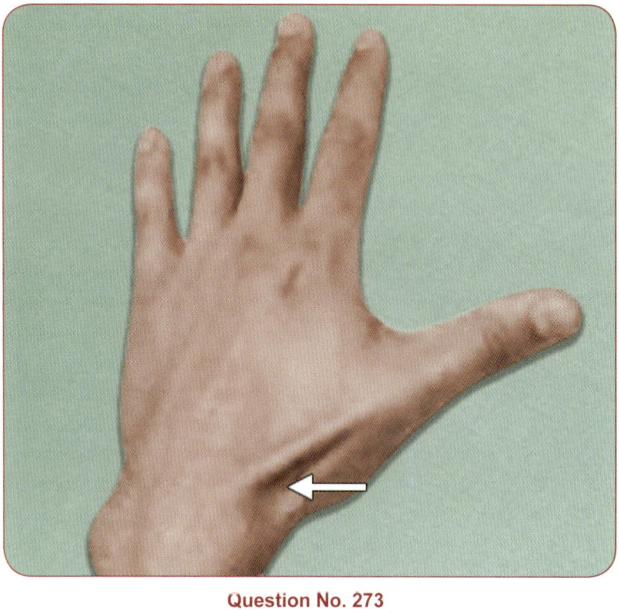

Question No. 273
Answer: Scaphoid

Plate 7

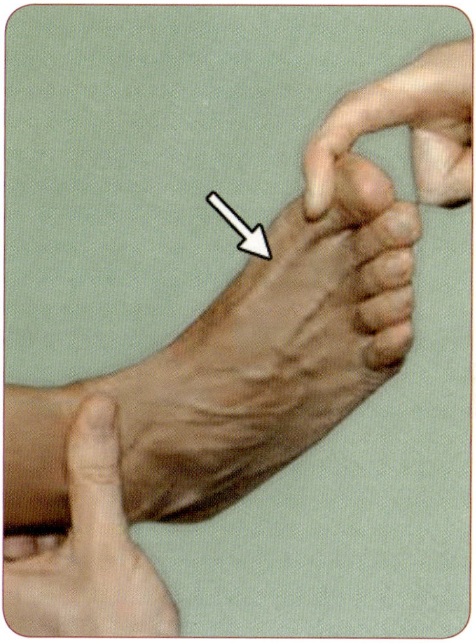

Question No. 274
Answer: Extensor hallucis longus

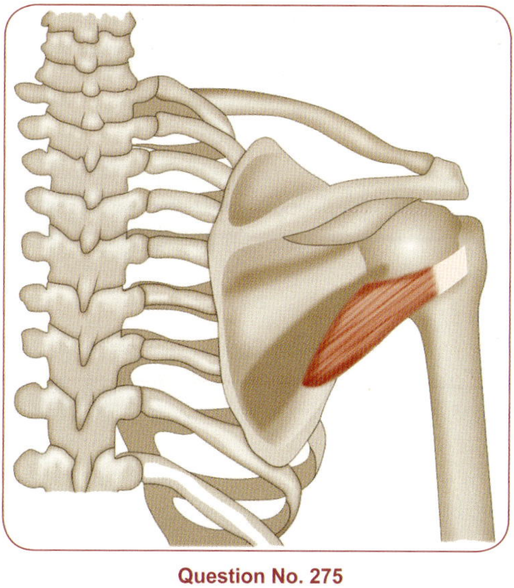

Question No. 275
Answer: Teres major

Plate 8

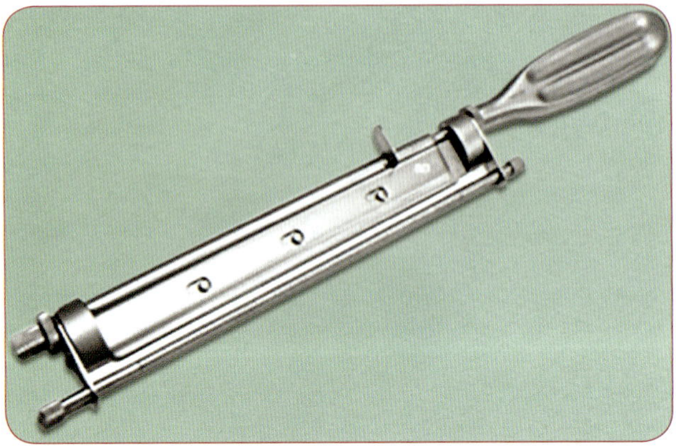

Question No. 276
Answer: Watson skin graft knife

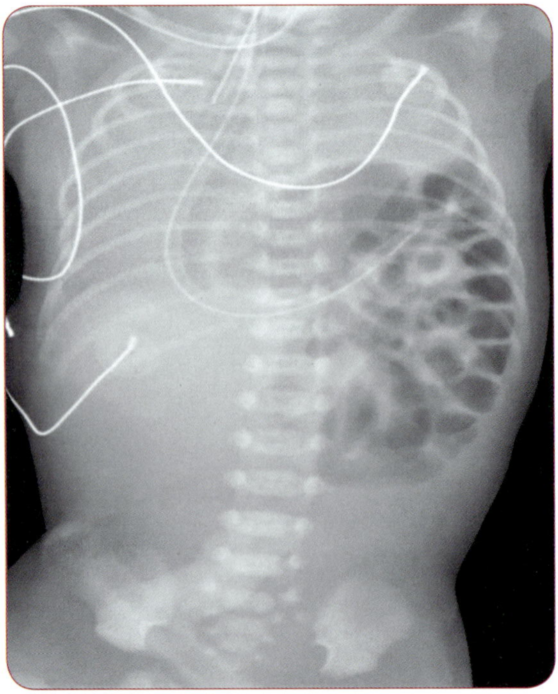

Question No. 277
Answer: Congenital diaphragmatic hernia

Plate 9

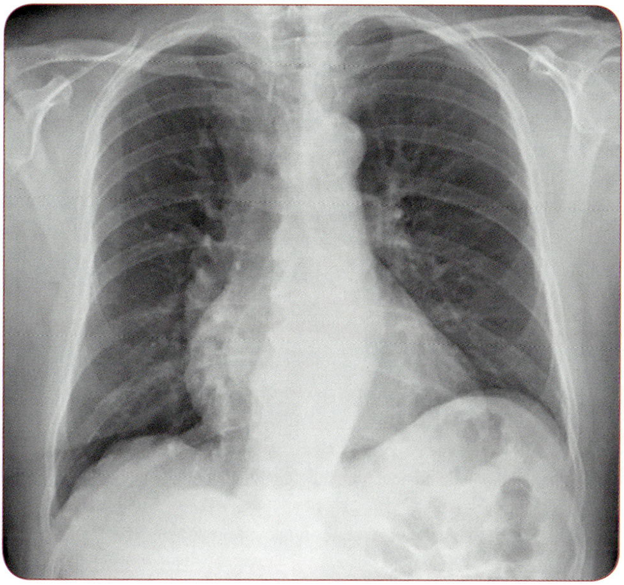

Question No. 278
Answer: Mitral stenosis

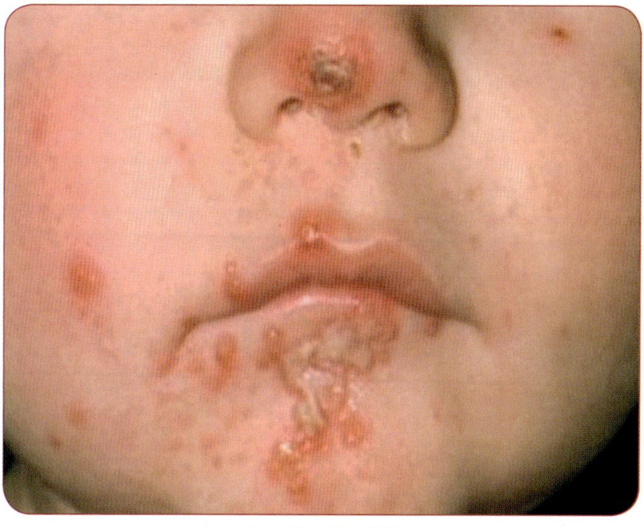

Question No. 279
Answer: Impetigo

Plate 10

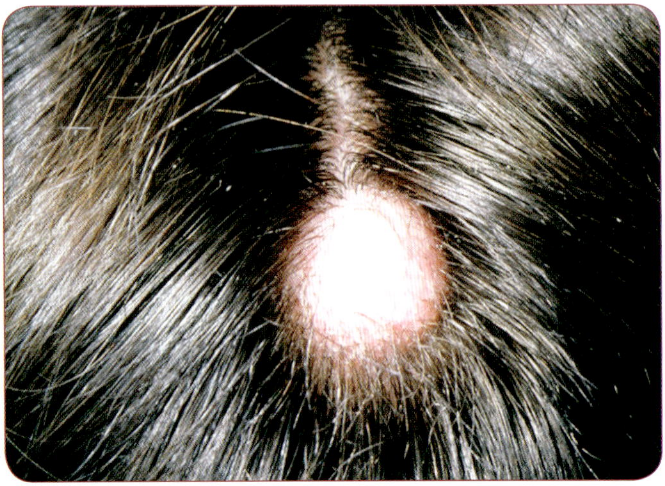

Question No. 280
Answer: Sebaceous cyst on scalp

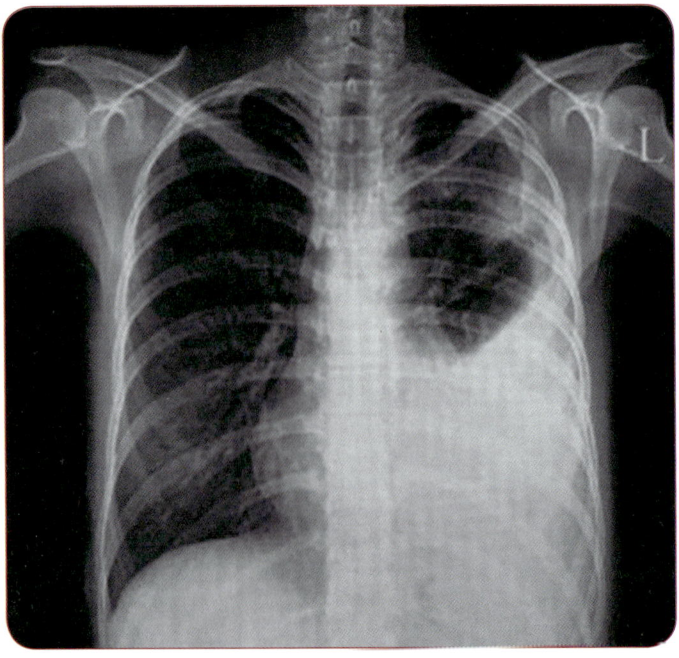

Question No. 281
Answer: Malignant pleural effusions

Plate 11

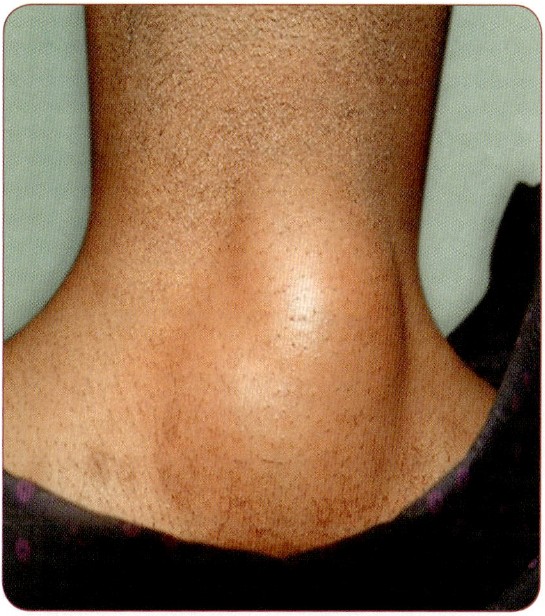

Question No. 282
Answer: Lipoma

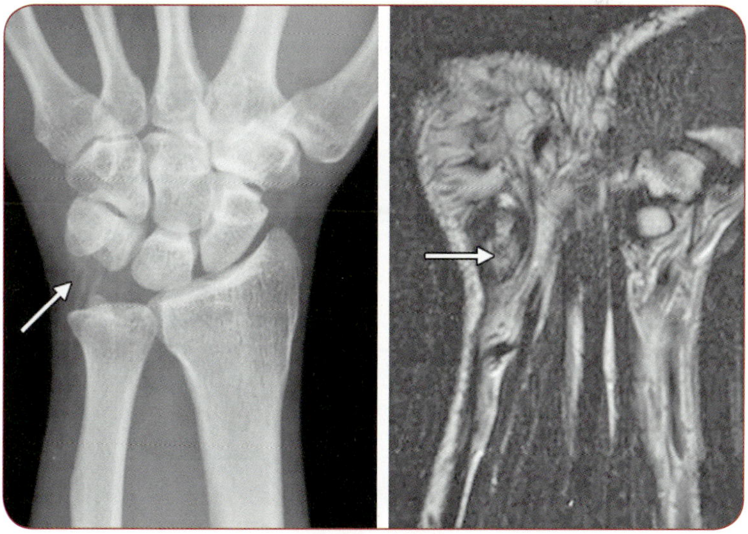

Question No. 283
Answer: Flexor carpi ulnaris

Plate 12

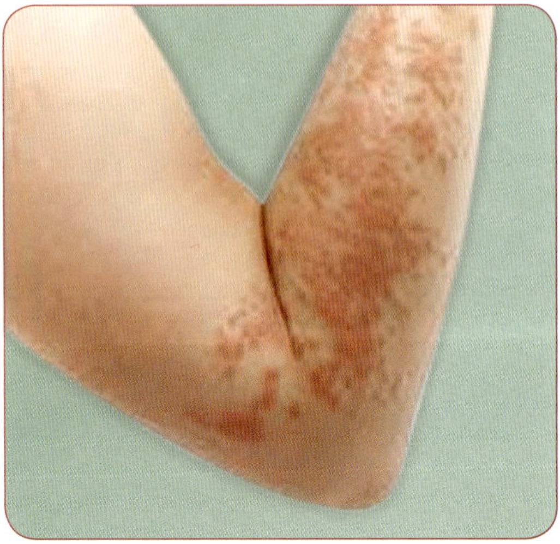

Question No. 284
Answer: Psoriasis

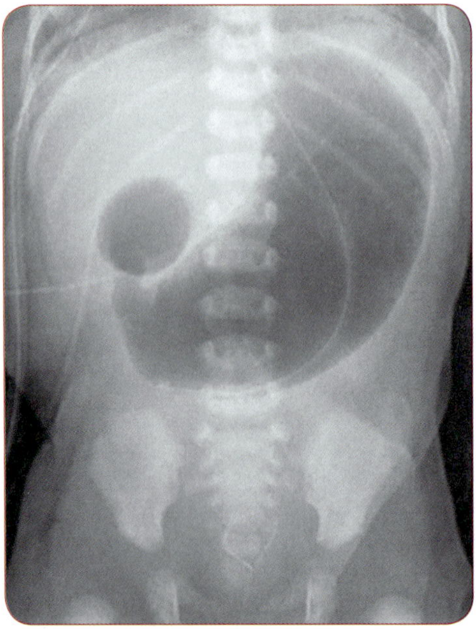

Question No. 285
Answer: Duodenal atresia

MCQs WITH EXPLANATIONS JUNE 2019

1. Which of the following is treatment chemoprophylaxis for *Cryptococcus*?

a. Fluconazole
b. Itraconazole
c. Ketaconazol
d. Oxiconazole

Ans. a. Fluconazole

(Ref: Essentials of Medical Pharmacology KDT 8th edition, page 232)

- Cryptococcosis that does not affect the central nervous system can be treated with fluconazole alone.
- Fluconazole is an antifungal medication used for a number of fungal infections. This includes candidiasis, blastomycosis, coccidiodomycosis, cryptococcosis, histoplasmosis, dermatophytosis, and pityriasis versicolor.
- It is also used to prevent candidiasis in those who are at high risk such as following organ transplantation, low birth weight babies, and those with low blood neutrophil counts. It is given either by mouth or by injection into a vein.

2. Erythema infectiosum is caused by which of the following?

a. Parvovirus
b. Adenoviruses
c. Herpesviruses
d. Poxviruses

Ans. a. Parvovirus

(Ref: Ananthanarayan and Paniker's Textbook of Microbiology 10th edition, page 332)

- Erythema infectiosum or fifth disease is one of several possible manifestations of infection by parvovirus B19.
- The name "fifth disease" comes from its place on the standard list of rash-causing childhood diseases, which also includes measles (first), scarlet fever (second), rubella (third), Dukes' disease (fourth, but is no longer widely accepted as distinct), and roseola (sixth).

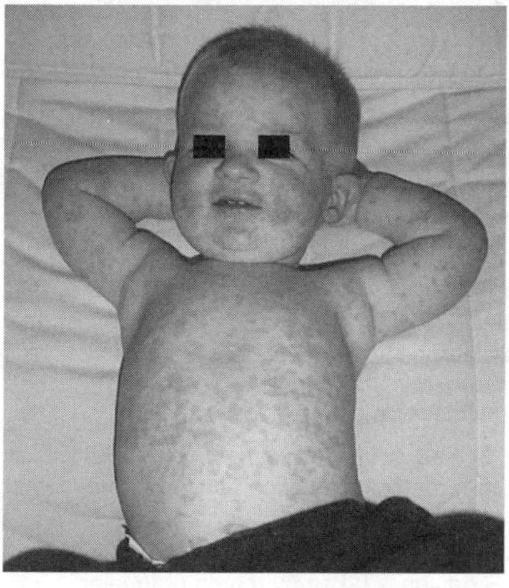

3. Which of the following conditions causes oligohydramnios?

a. Pelvic kidney
b. PKD
c. Renal agenesis
d. Renal ectopia

Ans. c. Renal agenesis *(Ref: Langman's Medical Embryology 11th edition, page 54)*

- Renal agenesis, Bilateral
- Synonyms of Renal Agenesis, Bilateral
  - Kidney Agenesis
  - Renal Agenesis

General Discussion

Bilateral renal agenesis is the absence of both kidneys at birth. It is a genetic disorder characterized by a failure of the kidneys to develop in a fetus. This absence of kidneys causes a deficiency of amniotic fluid (oligohydramnios) in a pregnant woman. Normally, the amniotic fluid acts as a cushion for the developing fetus. When there is an insufficient amount of this fluid, compression of the fetus may occur resulting in further malformations of the baby.

This disorder is more common in infants born of a parent who has a kidney malformation, particularly the absence of one kidney (unilateral renal agenesis). Studies have proven that unilateral renal agenesis and bilateral renal agenesis are genetically related.

Signs and Symptoms

Bilateral renal agenesis is characterized by the absence of kidneys and of urine in a baby. The face usually consists of wide-set eyes; a "parrot beak" nose; a receding chin, and large low set ears deficient in cartilage.

Potter sequence is the atypical physical appearance of a baby due to oligohydramnios experienced when in the uterus. It includes clubbed feet, pulmonary hypoplasia and cranial anomalies related to the oligohydramnios. Oligohydramnios is the decrease in amniotic fluid volume sufficient to cause deformations in morphogenesis of the baby.

4. Aerosol drug used for treatment of RSV infection in a child is:

a. Ribavirin
b. Amantadine
c. Indinavir
d. Tenofovir

Ans. a. Ribavirin *(Ref: Essentials of Medical Pharmacology KDT 8th edition, page 453)*

Ribavirin is an antiviral drug that was approved by the Food and Drug Administration (FDA) in 1986 for aerosol treatment of serious respiratory syncytial virus (RSV) infections in hospitalized children.

Ribavirin has a broad spectrum of antiviral activity in vitro, where it inhibits replication of RSV, influenza, parainfluenza, adenovirus, measles, Lassa fever, and Hantaan viruses. Proof of efficacy for human infection has been obtained in double-blind placebo-controlled studies of RSV, Lassa fever, and Korean hemorrhagic fever.

Ribavirin, also known as tribavirin, is an antiviral medication used to treat RSV infection, hepatitis C, and viral hemorrhagic fever. For hepatitis C, it is used in combination with other medications such as simeprevir, sofosbuvir, peginterferon alfa-2b or peginterferon alfa-2a. Among the viral hemorrhagic fevers it is used for Lassa fever, Crimean–Congo hemorrhagic fever, and Hantavirus infection but not Ebola or Marburg. Ribavirin is taken by mouth or inhaled.

5. Secretion of prolactin is inhibited by which of the following?

a. Adrenaline
b. Nor-adrenaline
c. Serotonin
d. Dopamine

Ans. d. Dopamine

(Ref: Guyton and Hall 13th edition, page 232)

Dopamine serves as the major prolactin-inhibiting factor or brake on prolactin secretion. Dopamine is secreted into portal blood by hypothalamic neurons, binds to receptors on lactotrophs, and inhibits both the synthesis and secretion of prolactin. Agents and drugs that interfere with dopamine secretion or receptor binding lead to enhanced secretion of prolactin.

In addition to tonic inhibition by dopamine, prolactin secretion is positively regulated by several hormones, including thyroid-releasing hormone, gonadotropin-releasing hormone and vasoactive intestinal polypeptide. Stimulation of the nipples and mammary gland, as occurs during nursing, leads to prolactin release. This effect appears to be due to a spinal reflex arc that causes release of prolactin-stimulating hormones from the hypothalamus.

In women the major action of prolactin is to initiate and sustain lactation. In breast-feeding mothers, tactile stimulation of the nipples and the breast by the suckling infant blocks the secretion of hypothalamic dopamine (which normally inhibits prolactin) into the hypophyseal-portal circulation of the pituitary gland. This results in a sharp rise in serum prolactin concentrations, followed by a prompt fall when feeding stops. High serum prolactin concentrations inhibit secretion of gonadotropin-releasing hormone (GnRH) from the hypothalamus, thereby decreasing the secretion of gonadotropins [luteinizing hormone (LH) and follicle-stimulating hormone (FSH)], and may also inhibit the action of gonadotropins on the gonads. Thus, high serum prolactin concentrations during lactation reduce fertility, protecting lactating women from a premature pregnancy.

6. Which of the following drug is a selective COX-2 inhibitor?

a. Etoricoxib
b. Ketorolac
c. Nimesulide
d. Piroxicam

Ans. a. Etorocoxib

(Ref: Essentials of Medical Pharmacology KDT 8th edition, page 325)

- Etoricoxib (Arcoxia) is a selective COX-2 inhibitor from Merck & Co. Currently it is approved in more than 80 countries worldwide but not in the US, where the FDA has required additional safety and efficacy data for etoricoxib before it will issue approval.
- It was patented in 1996 and approved for medical use in 2002.
- Some COX-2 inhibitors are used in a single dose to treat pain after surgery.
- Selective COX-2 inhibitors are a type of nonsteroidal anti-inflammatory drug (NSAID) that directly targets cyclo-oxygenase-2, COX-2, an enzyme responsible for inflammation and pain. Targeting selectivity for COX-2 reduces the risk of peptic ulceration, and is the main feature of celecoxib, rofecoxib and other members of this drug class.

7. Which of the following is a mood stabilizer?

a. Citalopram
b. Paroxetine
c. Escitalopram
d. Lithium

Ans. d. Lithium *(Ref: Essentials of Medical Pharmacology KDT 8th edition, page 431)*

Mood stabilizers represent a class of drugs that are efficacious in the treatment of bipolar disorder. The most established medications in this class are lithium, valproic acid, and carbamazepine. In addition to their therapeutic effects for treatment of acute manic episodes, these medications often are useful as prophylaxis against future episodes and as adjunctive antidepressant medications.

Which drugs are mood stabilizers?

The five individual drugs that can be used as mood stabilizers are:

- Lithium (Camcolit, Liskonum, Priadel, Lithonate, Litarex, Li-liquid)
- Carbamazepine (Tegretol)
- Lamotrigine (Lamictal)
- Valproate (Depakote, Epilim)
- Asenapine (Sycrest).

8. Which of the following is long acting broncho-dilator?

a. Terbutaline
b. Adrenaline
c. Formoterol
d. Salbutamol

Ans. c. Formoterol *(Ref: Essentials of Medical Pharmacology KDT 8th edition, page 126)*

Short-acting β-agonists: Such as salbutamol, are specific to the lungs; they are called β2-adrenergic agonists and can relieve bronchospasms without unwanted cardiac side effects of nonspecific β-agonists (e.g. ephedrine or epinephrine).

Long-acting β-agonists: These are long-term medications taken routinely in order to control and prevent bronchoconstriction.

Commonly taken twice a day with an anti-inflammatory medication, they maintain open airways and prevent asthma symptoms, particularly at night.

Salmeterol and formoterol are examples of these.

Anticholinergic: tiotropium (Spiriva) and ipratropium bromide.

Tiotropium is a long-acting, 24-hour, anticholinergic bronchodilator used in the management of chronic obstructive pulmonary disease (COPD).

9. Which of the following does not cause endometrial cancer?

a. Obesity
b. Diabetes
c. Hypothyroidism
d. Menopause

Ans. c. Hypothyroidism *(Ref: DC Dutta's Textbook of Obstetrics 9th edition, page 401)*

Endometrial cancer is cancer that starts in the endometrium, the lining of the uterus (womb).

Causes: Endometrial cancer is the most common type of uterine cancer. The exact cause of endometrial cancer is not known. An increased level of estrogen hormone may play a role. This stimulates the buildup of the lining of the uterus. This can lead to overgrowth of the endometrium and cancer.

Most cases of endometrial cancer occur between the ages of 60 and 70. A few cases may occur before age 40.

The following factors related to your hormones increase your risk for endometrial cancer:

- Estrogen replacement therapy without the use of progesterone
- History of endometrial polyps

- Infrequent periods
- Never being pregnant
- Obesity
- Diabetes
- Polycystic ovary syndrome (PCOS)
- Starting menstruation at an early age (before age 12)
- Starting menopause after age 50
- Tamoxifen, a drug used for breast cancer treatment.

Women with the following conditions also seem to be at a higher risk for endometrial cancer:

- Colon or breast cancer
- Gallbladder disease
- High blood pressure.

Endometrial cancer (EC) is one of the most common gynecological malignancies. Obesity, diabetes mellitus, hypertension, a continuous estrogen supply unopposed by progesterone, infertility, nulliparity, and tamoxifen use are widely accepted to be in involved in the pathogenesis of EC. Clinicians do not usually test the thyroid function of patients with EC, but, interestingly, hypothyroidism has been reported to be a common complication of EC, leading us to consider whether hypothyroidism is also a risk factor for EC. Currently, evidence on the direct relationship between hypothyroidism and EC is unavailable.

10. Healthy volunteers participate in which phase of clinical trial?

a. Phase 1 b. Phase 2
c. Phase 3 d. Phase 4

Ans. a. Phase 1

(Ref: Park's Textbook of Preventive and Social Medicine 25th edition, page 324)

Healthy volunteers in phase 1 clinical trials contribute to the development of safe drugs and other biologics and accept risks and burdens without anticipated health benefits from participation.

Although emerging data have shown that healthy volunteers are influenced by risk, some still worry that financial incentives lead them to take on unreasonable risk. Yet little is known about healthy volunteers' preferences and how they make choices about enrolling in research studies.

11. A patient presented with 3rd nerve palsy with contralateral hemiplegia. Which syndrome is this?

a. Weber's syndrome b. Lateral pontine syndrome
c. Medial medullary syndrome d. Medial pontine syndrome

Ans. a. Weber's syndrome *(Ref: Gray's Anatomy 41st edition, page 211)*

- Weber's syndrome, also known as superior alternating hemiplegia, is a form of stroke characterized by the presence of an ipsilateral oculomotor nerve palsy and contralateral hemiparesis or hemiplegia. It is caused by midbrain infarction as a result of occlusion of the paramedian branches of the posterior cerebral artery or of basilar bifurcation perforating arteries.
- It is caused by midbrain infarction as a result of occlusion of the paramedian branches of the posterior cerebral artery or of basilar bifurcation perforating arteries.

- Clinical findings mainly eyeball is down and out ipsilateral lateral squint. Ptosis present. Pupil dilated and fixed as lipopolysaccharide (LPS) nerve supply is disrupted. Contralateral hemiplegia CT scan or MRI might help in delineating the cause or the vessel or region of brain involved in stroke.

12. Treatment of keloid:

a. Intralesional triamcinolone acetonide
b. Radiotherapy
c. Anti-metabolites
d. Corticoids

Ans. a. Intralesional triamcinolone acetonide

(Ref: Bailey & Love's Short Practice of Surgery, 27th edition, page 219)

The best treatment is prevention in patients with a known predisposition. This includes preventing unnecessary trauma or surgery (including ear piercing, elective mole removal), whenever possible. Any skin problems in predisposed individuals (e.g. acne, infections) should be treated as early as possible to minimize areas of inflammation.

Treatment of a keloid scar is age dependent. Radiotherapy, anti-metabolites and corticoids would not be recommended to be used in children, in order to avoid harmful side effects, like growth abnormalities.

In adults, corticosteriods combined with 5-FU and PDL in a triple therapy, enhance results and diminish side effects.

Further prophylactic and therapeutic strategies include pressure therapy, silicone gel sheeting, intralesional triamcinolone acetonide (TAC), cryosurgery, radiation, laser therapy, IFN, 5-FU and surgical excision as well as a multitude of extracts and topical agents.

13. Triple test for Down syndrome consists of all *except*:

a. AFP
b. Estriol
c. Beta HCG
d. Inhibin alpha

Ans. d. Inhibin alpha *(Ref: DC Dutta's Textbook of Obstetrics 9th edition, page 341)*

The triple test measures the following three levels in the maternal serum:

1. Alpha-fetoprotein (AFP)
2. Human chorionic gonadotropin (hCG)
3. Unconjugated estriol (UE3)

The triple test, also called triple screen, the Kettering test or the Bart's test, is an investigation performed during pregnancy in the second trimester to classify a patient as either high-risk or low-risk for chromosomal abnormalities (and neural tube defects).

The most common abnormality the test can screen is trisomy 21 (Down syndrome). In addition to Down syndrome, the triple and quadruple screens assess risk for fetal trisomy 18 also known as Edward's syndrome, open neural tube defects, and may also detect an increased risk of Turner syndrome, triploidy, trisomy 16 mosaicism, fetal death, Smith–Lemli–Opitz syndrome, and steroid sulfatase deficiency.

Quadruple Test

A test of levels of dimeric inhibin A (DIA) is sometimes added to the other three tests, under the name "quadruple test".

Other names used include "quad test", "quad screen", or "tetra screen." Inhibin A will be found high in cases of trisomy 21 and low in cases of trisomy 18.

Inhibin A	Associated conditions
High	Trisomy 21 (Down syndrome)
Low	Trisomy 18 (Edwards syndrome)
Variable	Trisomy 13 (Patau syndrome)

14. Jaundice is clinically visible when bilirubin level is more than:

a. >3 mg/dL b. >0.5 mg/dL
c. >1 mg/dL d. >2 mg/dL

Ans. a. >3 mg/dL *(Ref: Guyton and Hall 13th edition, page 209)*

- Causes of jaundice vary from non-serious to potentially fatal. Levels of bilirubin in blood are normally below 1.0 mg/dL (17 µmol/L) and levels over 2–3 mg/dL (34–51 µmol/L) typically results in jaundice.
- High bilirubin is divided into two types: (1) unconjugated (indirect) and (2) conjugated (direct).
- The main sign of jaundice is a yellowish discoloration of the white area of the eye and the skin.
- Urine is dark in color. Slight increases in serum bilirubin are best detected by examining the sclera, which have a particular affinity for bilirubin due to their high elastin content.
- The presence of scleral icterus indicates a serum bilirubin of at least 3 mg/dL.

15. Greenish color in putrefaction is due to formation of:

a. Sulfhemoglobinemia b. Methemoglobinemia
c. Carboxyhemoglobinemia d. Oxyhaemoglobin

Ans. a. Sulfhemoglobinemia *(Ref: Robbins Basic Pathology 10th edition, page 675)*

Sulfhemoglobinemia is a rare condition in which there is excess sulfhemoglobin (SulfHb) in the blood. The pigment is a greenish derivative of hemoglobin which cannot be converted back to normal, functional hemoglobin. It causes cyanosis even at low blood levels.

It is a rare blood condition that occurs when a sulfur atom is incorporated into the hemoglobin molecule. When hydrogen sulfide (H_2S) (or sulfide ions) and ferric ions combine in the blood, the blood is incapable of carrying oxygen.

16. Management of olecranon fracture:

a. Tension band wiring b. Intramedullary fixation and plates
c. Excision d. Triceps advancement

Ans. a. Tension band wiring

(Ref: Rockwood and Green's Fractures in Adults 8th edition, page 33)

Olecranon fracture is a fracture of the bony portion of the elbow. The injury is fairly common and often occurs following a fall or direct trauma to the elbow. The olecranon is the proximal extremity of the ulna which is articulated with the humerus bone and constitutes a part of the elbow articulation. Its location makes it vulnerable to direct trauma.

- **Displaced fractures:** Most olecranon fractures are displaced and are best treated surgically.
- **Tension band fixation:** Tension band fixation is the most common form of internal fixation used for non-comminuted olectranon fractures. It is typically reserved for noncomminuted fractures that are proximal to the coronoid. This procedure is performed using Kirschner wire (K-wires) which converts tensile forces into compressive force.
- **Intramedullary fixation and plates:** Single intramedullary screws can be used to treat simple transverse or oblique fractures. Plates can be used for all proximal ulna fracture types including Monteggia fractures, and comminuted fractures.
- **Excision and triceps advancement:** This method is indicated for cases when open reduction and internal fixation is unlikely to be successful. For example, extensive comminutions, elderly patients with osteoporotic bone, and small or non-union fractures.

17. Which of the following is done to study the prevalence?

a. Cohort study b. Cross-sectional study
c. Case-control studies d. Panel study

Ans. b. Cross-sectional study

(Ref: Park's Textbook of Preventive & Social Medicine 25th edition, page 329)

A cross-sectional study (also known as a cross-sectional analysis, transverse study, prevalence study) is a type of observational study that analyzes data from a population, or a representative subset, at a specific point in time—i.e. cross-sectional data.

In medical research, cross-sectional studies differ from case-control studies in that they aim to provide data on the entire population under study, whereas case-control studies typically include only individuals with a specific characteristic, with a sample, often a tiny minority, of the rest of the population. Cross-sectional studies are descriptive studies (neither longitudinal nor experimental). Unlike case-control studies, they can be used to describe, not only the odds ratio, but also absolute risks and relative risks from prevalences (sometimes called prevalence risk ratio, or PRR).

They may be used to describe some feature of the population, such as prevalence of an illness, or they may support inferences of cause and effect. Longitudinal studies differ from both in making a series of observations more than once on members of the study population over a period of time.

18. Most common part affected in intestinal TB is:

a. Ileocecal region b. Esophagus
c. Stomach d. Colon

Ans. a. Ileocecal region *(Ref: Robbins Basic Pathology 10th edition, page 430)*

- The most common site of the gastrointestinal TB is ileocecal location (ileocecal TB), followed by jejunum and colon. The esophagus, stomach and duodenum are rarely involved.
- The most common site of involvement of the gastrointestinal tuberculosis is the ileocaecal region. Ileocaecal and small bowel tuberculosis presents with a palpable mass in the right lower quadrant and/or complications of obstruction, perforation or malabsorption especially in the presence of stricture.

19. Color of nitrous oxide cylinder is:

a. White
b. Black
c. Blue
d. Blue body with white shoulder

Ans. c. Blue *(Ref: Morgan and Mikhail's Clinical Anesthesiology, 6th edition, Page 239)*

Gas	USA	International
Oxygen	Green	White
Carbon dioxide	Gray	Gray
Nitrous oxide	Blue	Blue
Helium	Brown	Brown
Nitrogen	Black	Black
Air	Yellow	White and black

Nitrous oxide, commonly known as laughing gas or nitrous, is a chemical compound an oxide of nitrogen with the formula N_2O. At room temperature, it is a colorless non-flammable gas, with a slightly metallic scent and taste. At elevated temperatures, nitrous oxide is a powerful oxidizer similar to molecular oxygen. The cylinders used to store the nitrous oxide are of blue color.

20. Drug of choice for treatment of Alzheimer's disease:

a. Atropine
b. Donepezil
c. Fluoxetine
d. Physostigmine

Ans. b. Donepezil *(Ref: Essentials of Medical Pharmacology KDT 8th edition, page 651)*

Treatment of choice	
1. Erythrodermic psoriasis	Methotrexate
2. Psoriatic arthropathy	• Methotrexate
3. Severe erythrodermic psoriasis	Cyclosporine
4. Pustular psoriasis	Acitretin (Retinoid)
5. Impetigo herpetiformis	Systemic steroids
6. Arthritis mutilans	Etanercept
7. Guttate psoriasis	Macrolide
8. Genital warts imiquimod	• Podophyllin (CI in pregnancy)
9. Genital warts in pregnancy	Cryotherapy > Trichloroacetic acid
10. Syphilis	Benzathine penicillin 2.4 million units
11. Neurosyphilis	Aqueous penicillin
12. Herpes	Acyclovir or foscarnet
13. Donovanosis	Azithromycin or doxycycline
14. LGV	Doxycycline or tetracycline
15. Chancroid	Ceftriaxone > Azithromycin

Contd...

Contd…

Treatment of choice	
16. *Neisseria*	Ceftriaxone
17. *Cryptococcus*	Induction: Amphotericin maintenance: Fluconazole
18. *Pneumocystis carinii*	Cotrimoxazole* 14d (21d in HIV)
19. Invasive aspergillosis	Voriconazole
20. Aspergillosis	Itraconazole
21. *Sporothrix*	Itraconazole
22. Blastomycosis	Amphotericin B
23. Coccidioidomycosis	Itraconazole
24. Paracoccidioidomycosis	Itraconazole
25. Dermatitis herpetiformis	Gluten free diet > Dapsone (DOC)
26. Pemphigus vulgaris	Prednisolone
27. Porphyria cutanea tarda	Venesection > Low dose chloroquine
28. Xerostomia	Cevimeline (muscarinic agonist)
29. Atropine (*Belladonna* poison)	Physostigmine
30. Alzheimer's disease	Donepezil (Tertiary carbamate)
31. Diagnosis of myasthenia	Edrophonium
32. Myasthenia gravis	Pyridostigmine
33. Open angle glaucoma	Prostaglandins analogs

Drug agent	Doc for
Streptomycin	1. Tularemia
Oseltamivir	2. Influenza
Tetracaine	3. Spinal anesthesia
Amytriptyline	4. Multiple sclerosis
Betaxolol	5. Emergency HTN beta blocker
Oxytocin	6. Postpartum hemorrhage
Neostigmine	7. Myasthenia gravis
Promethazine	8. Delayed HTNivity reaction
Levodopa	9. Parkinsons
Codeine	10. Dry itchy cough
Chloramphenicol	11. Typhoid fever
Vancomycin	12. Pseudomembranous colitis
Acyclovir	13. Herpes
Metronidazole	14. Trichomoniasis
Lithium carbonate	15. Mania
Omeprazole	16. Peptic ulcer
ORS	17. Mainstay for diarrhea
Diazepam	18. Status epilepticus

Contd…

Contd...

Drug agent	Doc for
Phenobarbital	19. Status epilepticus in children
Oxytocin	20. Postpartum breast engorgement
Belladonna	21. Neostigmine induced diarrhea
Epinephrine	22. Anaphylactic shock
Ergotamine	23. Migraine
Ferrous sulfate	24. Microcytic anemia
Carbon dioxide	25. Persistent hiccups
Ipratropium bromide	26. Bronchospasm with COPD
Imipramine	27. Enuresis
Tegaserod	28. Constipation due to IBS in women
Misoprostol	29. GI ulceration
Mannitol	30. Cerebral edema
Mannitol	31. Intracranial pressure
Diuretic	32. Mild HTN
Carbamazepine	33. Psychomotor seizure
Mupirocin	34. Impetigo
Nitroprusside	35. Hypertensive crisis
Carbamazepine	36. Trigeminal neuralgia

21. Mechanism of action of atropine in treatment of organophosphate poisoning is:

a. It inhibits secretion of acetylcholine
b. It is re-activator of acetylcholine esterase enzyme
c. It is agonist of acetylcholine receptors
d. It has antimuscarinic activity

Ans. d. It has antimuscarinic activity

(Ref: Essentials of Medical Pharmacology KDT 8th edition, page 341)

- Atropine can be used as an antidote in conjunction with pralidoxime or other pyridinium oximes (such as trimedoxime or obidoxime), though the use of "-oximes" has been found to be of no benefit, or to be possibly harmful, in at least two meta-analyses.
- Atropine is a muscarinic antagonist, and thus blocks the action of acetylcholine peripherally.
- In general, atropine counters the "rest and digest" activity of glands regulated by the parasympathetic nervous system. This occurs because atropine is a competitive, reversible antagonist of the muscarinic acetylcholine receptors (acetylcholine being the main neurotransmitter used by the parasympathetic nervous system).
- Atropine is a competitive antagonist of the muscarinic acetylcholine receptor types M1, M2, M3, M4 and M5. It is classified as an anticholinergic drug (parasympatholytic).

22. Drug of choice for neurogenic diabetes insipidus is:

a. Vasopressin
b. Desmopressin
c. Terlipressin
d. Conivaptan

Ans. b. Desmopressin

(Ref: Harrison's Principles of Internal Medicine 20th edition vol 1, page 231)

- The disorder is treated with vasopressin analogs such as desmopressin. Nonetheless, many times desmopressin alone is not enough to bring under control all the symptoms, and another intervention must be implemented.
- Central diabetes insipidus, also called neurogenic diabetes insipidus, is a type of diabetes insipidus due to a lack of vasopressin (ADH) production in the brain. Vasopressin acts to increase the volume of blood (intravascularly), and decrease the volume of urine produced. Therefore, a lack of it causes increased urine production and volume depletion.
- It is also known as neurohypophyseal diabetes insipidus, referring to the posterior pituitary (neurohypophysis), which is supplied by the hypothalamus in the brain.

23. Which of the following inhalational anesthetic agent can cause hepatitis on repeated use?

a. Ether
b. Halothane
c. Isoflurane
d. Sevoflurane

Ans. b. Halothane

(Ref: Morgan and Mikhail's Clinical Anesthesiology, 6th edition, page 231)

- Repeated exposure to halothane in adults was noted to result in severe liver injury. This occurred in about one in 10,000 exposures.
- The resulting syndrome was referred to as halothane hepatitis, and is thought to result from the metabolism of halothane to trifluoroacetic acid via oxidative reactions in the liver.
- About 20% of inhaled halothane is metabolized by the liver and these products are excreted in the urine. The hepatitis syndrome had a mortality rate of 30% to 70%.
- Concern for hepatitis resulted in a dramatic reduction in the use of halothane for adults and it was replaced in the 1980s by enfluraneand isoflurane. By 2005, the most common volatile anesthetics used were is oflurane, sevoflurane, and desflurane.

24. Preferred drug for the treatment of ventricular tachycardia is:

a. Lignocaine
b. Diltiazem
c. Digoxin
d. Propranolol

Ans. a. Lignocaine

(Ref: Harrison's Principles of Internal Medicine 20th edition vol 1, page 433)

- Lidocaine, also known as lignocaine, is a medication used to numb tissue in a specific area (local anesthetic). It is also used to treat ventricular tachycardia and to perform nerve blocks.
- Lidocaine is also the most important class-1b antiarrhythmic drug; it is used intravenously for the treatment of ventricular arrhythmias (for acute myocardial infarction, digoxin poisoning, cardioversion, or cardiac catheterization) if amiodarone is not available or contraindicated.

- Lidocaine should be given for this indication after defibrillation, Cardiopulmonary resuscitation (CPR), and vasopressors have been initiated. A routine preventative dose is no longer recommended after a myocardial infarction as the overall benefit is not convincing.

25. Drug of choice for chronic gout is:

a. Febuxostat
b. Probenecid
c. Allopurinol
d. Sulfinpyrazone

Ans. c. Allopurinol

(Ref: Harrison's Principles of Internal Medicine 20th edition vol 1, page 521)

- Allopurinol is used to reduce urate formation in conditions where urate deposition has already occurred or is predictable.
- The specific diseases and conditions where it is used include gouty arthritis, skin tophi, kidney stones, idiopathic gout; uric acid lithiasis; acute uric acid nephropathy; neoplastic disease and myeloproliferative disease with high cell turnover rates, in which high urate levels occur either spontaneously, or after cytotoxic therapy; certain enzyme disorders which lead to overproduction of urate, e.g. hypoxanthine-guanine phosphoribosyltransferase, including Lesch–Nyhan syndrome; glucose 6-phosphatase including glycogen storage disease; phosphoribosyl pyrophosphate synthetase, phosphoribosyl pyrophosphate amidotransferase; adenine phosphoribosyltransferase.
- It is also used to treat kidney stones caused by deficient activity of adenine phosphoribosyltransferase.

26. Which of the following is use for day care surgery?

a. Ketamine
b. Propofol
c. Etomidate
d. Thiopentone

Ans. b. Propofol

(Ref: Morgan and Mikhail's Clinical Anesthesiology, 6th edition, page 236)

- Anesthesia of a choice for day care surgery, short acting action diminishes the same day. Propofol (25–50 mcg/kg/min) is the most commonly used drug for induction of anesthesia, maintenance of sedation and treatment of nausea and vomiting.
- Thiopentone, etomidate, and ketamine have been used, but now mostly replaced by Propofol. Etomidate (0.2–0.3 mg/kg) is preferred when hemodynamic stability is important.

27. A female with 20 weeks pregnancy present with fever and dysuria. A preliminary diagnosis of cystitis was made. Which of the following drugs will be safe to use for this patient?

a. Amoxicillin
b. Gentamicin
c. Ciprofloxacin
d. Cotrimoxazole

Ans. a. Amoxicillin *(Ref: DC Dutta's Textbook of Obstetrics 9th edition, page 763)*

- A urinary tract infection (UTI) is an infection that affects part of the urinary tract. When it affects the lower urinary tract it is known as a bladder infection (cystitis) and when it affects the upper urinary tract it is known as a kidney infection (pyelonephritis)

- Amoxicillin/clavulanic acid is widely used to treat or prevent many infections caused by susceptible bacteria, such as:
    - Urinary tract infections
    - Respiratory tract infections
    - Skin and soft tissue infections
    - Sinus infections
    - Cat scratches
    - Infections caused by the bacterial flora of the mouth, such as:
        - Dental infections
        - Infected animal bites
        - Infected human bites (including uncomplicated "clenched-fist" or "reverse-bite" injuries).
- This combination results in an antibiotic with an increased spectrum of action and restored efficacy against amoxicillin-resistant bacteria that produce β-lactamase.

28. Insulin of choice for the treatment of diabetes mellitus:

a. NPH insulin
b. Insulin glargine
c. Insulin lispro
d. Regular insulin

Ans. d. Regular insulin

(Ref: Harrison's Principles of Internal Medicine 20th edition vol 1, page 630)

- There are a number of different classes of anti-diabetic medications. Some are available by mouth, such as metformin, while others are only available by injection such as GLP-1 agonists.
- Type 1 diabetes can only be treated with insulin, typically with a combination of regular and NPH insulin, or synthetic insulin analogs.

29. Anti depressant drug which is used for smoking cessation is:

a. Bupropion
b. Amitriptyline
c. Venlafaxine
d. Topiramate

Ans. a. Bupropion

(Ref: Essentials of Medical Pharmacology KDT 8th edition, page 328)

- Bupropion is a pill that may cut down your craving for tobacco.
- Bupropion is also used for people with depression. It helps with quitting tobacco even if you do not have problems with depression.
- It is not fully clear how bupropion helps with tobacco cravings and quitting tobacco.

Bupropion should not be used for people who:

- Are under age 18
- Are pregnant
- Have a history of medical problems such seizures, kidney failure, heavy alcohol use, eating disorders, bipolar or manic depressive illness, or a serious head injury.

30. Praziquental is used for the treatment of:

a. Strongyloidiasis
b. Trichomoniasis
c. Rhinosporidoisis
d. Schistosomiasis

Ans. d. Schistosomiasis

(Ref: Essentials of Medical Pharmacology KDT 8th edition, page 400)

There are two drugs available, praziquantel and oxamniquine, for the treatment of schistosomiasis. They are considered equivalent in relation to efficacy against S. mansoni and safety. Because of praziquantel's lower cost per treatment, and oxaminiquine's lack of efficacy against the urogenital form of the disease caused by *S. haematobium*, in general praziquantel is considered the first option for treatment.

The treatment objective is to cure the disease and to prevent the evolution of the acute to the chronic form of the disease. All cases of suspected schistosomiasis should be treated regardless of presentation because the adult parasite can live in the host for years.

Schistosomiasis is treatable by taking by mouth a single dose of the drug praziquantel annually.

31. A young male present with reduce sleep, hyperactivity and elevated mood. He has a family history of mania. Which of the following drug should be used for long term treatment of this patient?

a. Lithium carbonate
b. Barbiturates
c. Sodium valproate
d. Carbamazepine

Ans. a. Lithium carbonate

(Ref: Harrison's Principles of Internal Medicine 20th edition, vol 1, page 387)

- Lithium carbonate is used to treat mania, the elevated phase of bipolar disorder. Lithium ions interfere with ion transport processes (*see* "sodium pump") that relay and amplify messages carried to the cells of the brain.
- Mania is associated with irregular increases in protein kinase C (PKC) activity within the brain. Lithium carbonate and sodium valproate, another drug traditionally used to treat the disorder, act in the brain by inhibiting PKC's activity and help to produce other compounds that also inhibit the PKC.
- Lithium carbonate's mood-controlling properties are not fully understood.

32. Shortest acting corticosteroid among the following:

a. Dexamethasone
b. Hydrocortisone
c. Deflazacort
d. Triamcinolone

Ans. b. Hydrocortisone

(Ref: Harrison's Principles of Internal Medicine 20th edition, vol 2, page 602)

Corticosteroid	Activity	Relative potency	Equivalent dose (mg)
Dexamethasone	Long-acting	25	0.75
Prednisone	Intermediate-acting	4	5.0
Methylprednisolone	Intermediate-acting	5	4.0
Hydrocortisone	Short-acting	1.0	20.0

33. Long-term use of which of the following drug is most likely associated with development of tremors?

a. Timolol
b. Betaxolol
c. Propofol
d. Salbutamol

Ans. d. Salbutamol

(Ref: Harrison's Principles of Internal Medicine 20th edition, vol 2, page 209)

- Tremor, a salbutamol induced tremor can either be long-term or short-term and occurs in 2–4% of regular salbutamol takers.
- The tremor is dose-related, and the theory of why it causes the tremor is still unexplained.
- However, the initial understanding suggests that the B2 adrenoreceptor agonist (salbutamol) has a direct effect on the muscles active state this' leads to incomplete fusion and reduced tension of tetanic contractions. More recently, tremor has been correlated closely with hypokalaemia.
- Increased pulse and tolerance are the main side effects of using salbutamol.

34. Which of the following anti-epileptic drug has highest teratogenic potential?

a. Valproate
b. Carbamazepine
c. Phenytoin
d. Lamotrigine

Ans. a. Valproate

(Ref: Harrison's Principles of Internal Medicine 20th edition, vol 1, page 285)

- The drug is known to cause serious abnormalities in the baby if taken during pregnancy. Because of this it is not typically recommended in women of childbearing age who have migraines
- Most recently, the Neurodevelopmental Effects of Antiepileptic Drugs (NEAD) Study Group confirmed both the increased risk of poor fetal outcome (MCM or death) and the dose-dependent effect of VPA in a prospective study (20.3% with VPA vs 10.7% with PHT, 8.2% with CBZ and 1% with LMT).

35. Abductor of hip joint:

a. Gluteus medius
b. Gluteus Maximus
c. Gluteus Minimus
d. Sartorius

Ans. a. Gluteus medius *(Ref: Gray's Anatomy 41st edition, page 306)*

Gluteus medius

- The anterior part acting alone helps to flex and internally rotate the hip.
- The posterior part acting alone helps to extend and externally rotate the hip.
- The anterior and posterior parts working together abduct the hip and stabilize the pelvis in the coronal plane.

Gluteus maximus (also known collectively with the gluteus medius and minimus, as the gluteal muscles, and sometimes referred to informally as the "glutes") is the main extensor muscle of the hip.

36. Adduction, flexion and medial rotation at shoulder joint is by which muscle?

a. Pectoralis major
b. Pectoralis minor
c. Teres major
d. Triceps brachii

Ans. a. Pectoralis major

(Ref: Gray's Anatomy 41st edition, page 426)

Pectoralis major: The pectoralis major has four actions which are primarily responsible for movement of the shoulder joint. The first action is flexion of the humerus, as in throwing a ball underhand, and in lifting a child. Secondly, it adducts the humerus, as when flapping the arms. Thirdly, it rotates the humerus medially, as occurs when arm-wrestling. Fourthly the pectoralis major is also responsible for keeping the arm attached to the trunk of the body.

Infraspinatus: This rotator cuff muscle helps with the raising and lowering of the upper arm.

Triceps brachii: This large muscle in the back of the upper arm helps straighten the arm.

Pectoralis minor: The smaller of the pectoralis muscles, this muscle fans out from the upper ribs up to the shoulder area.

Teres major: This muscle helps rotate the upper arm.

Biceps brachii: Commonly known as the bicep muscle, this muscle rests on top of the humerus bone. It rotates the forearm and also flexes the elbow.

Latissimus dorsi: This flat rectangular muscle of the back helps the arms rotate as well as move away and closer to the body.

Subscapularis: This is a large triangular muscle near the humerus and collarbone. It helps rotate the humerus.

Supraspinatus: This small muscle is located at the top of the shoulder and helps raise the arm away from the body.

37. Inferior angle of scapula lies at which vertebral level?

a. Opposite spinous process of T7
b. L1 or 2 vertebral level
c. T3 vertebra
d. Opposite the T10 vertebra

Ans. a. Opposite spinous process of T7

(Ref: Gray's Anatomy 41st edition, page 423)

- The vertebral levels summarized below are useful. The spinous processes of the C6 and 7 and T1 vertebra are usually visible in vivo when the neck is flexed.
- The apex of the lung and the cupola of the pleura extend to the C7 vertebral level.
- The spine of the scapula is commonly in line with the T3 vertebra, and the manubrium of the sternum is generally opposite T3 and 4 vertebrae.
- The trachea divides at the level of vertebrae T5 to 7 when a subject is in the erect position. The inferior angle of the scapula is frequently at the level of the spinous process of the T7 vertebra.
- The xiphisternal junction is approximately opposite the T10 vertebra.
- The spinal cord usually ends at the L1 or 2 vertebral level. The supracristal plane (through the highest points of the iliac crests), which is typically at the L4 vertebral level, is used as a landmark for lumbar puncture, and the aorta divides at this level.
- The anterior and posterior superior iliac spines (the latter being frequently marked by a dimple) are at the level of the second sacral segment.

38. Upper lateral cutaneous nerve of arm is a branch of:

a. Axillary nerve
b. Radial nerve
c. Musculocutaneous nerve
d. Median nerve

Ans. a. Axillary nerve *(Ref: Gray's Anatomy 41st edition, page 62)*

The superior lateral cutaneous nerve of arm (or superior lateral brachial cutaneous nerve) is the continuation of the posterior cord of the axillary nerve, after it pierces the deep fascia.

39. Testicular artery is a branch of:

a. Abdominal aorta
b. Inferior epigastric artery
c. External iliac artery
d. Internal iliac artery

Ans. a. Abdominal aorta *(Ref: Gray's Anatomy 41st edition, page 653)*

- The testicular artery (the male gonadal artery, also called the internal spermatic arteries in older texts) is a branch of the abdominal aorta that supplies blood to the testis. It is a paired artery, with one for each of the testes.
- It is the male equivalent of the ovarian artery. Because the testis is found in a different location than that of its female equivalent, it has a different course than the ovarian artery.
- They are two slender vessels of considerable length, and arise from the front of the aorta a little below the renal arteries.
- Each passes obliquely downward and lateralward behind the peritoneum, resting on the Psoas major, the right lying in front of the inferior vena cava and behind the middle colic and ileocolic arteries and the terminal part of the ileum, the left behind the left colic and sigmoid arteries and the iliac colon.
- Each crosses obliquely over the ureter and the lower part of the external iliac artery to reach the abdominal inguinal ring, through which it passes, and accompanies the other constituents of the spermatic cord along the inguinal canal to the scrotum, where it becomes tortuous, and divides into several branches.
- Two or three of these accompany the ductus deferens, and supply the epididymis, anastomosing with the artery of the ductus deferens; others pierce the back part of the tunica albuginea, and supply the substance of the testis.
- The internal spermatic artery supplies one or two small branches to the ureter, and in the inguinal canal gives one or two twigs to the cremaster.

40. A patient with hypothenar muscle wasting and loss of sensation on little finger and medial half of ring finger. Which nerve is involved?

a. Ulnar nerve
b. Median nerve
c. Radial nerve
d. Axillary nerve

Ans. a. Ulnar nerve

(Ref: Gray's Anatomy 41st edition, page 541)

While the exact cause of ulnar neuritis is unknown, there are several factors that can cause pressure on the ulnar nerve:

- The ulnar nerve constantly sliding back and forth from the medial epicondyle can irritate the nerve.
- Applying pressure to the elbow for long periods of time.
- Fluid buildup in the elbow causing swelling.
- A direct blow to the inside of the elbow can cause pain, electric shock sensation, and numbness in the little and ring fingers. This is commonly called "hitting your funny bone".

- Prior fracture or dislocations of the elbow.
- Bone spurs/arthritis of the elbow.
- Swelling of the elbow joint.
- Cysts near the elbow joint.
- Repetitive or prolonged activities where the elbow to be bent or flexed.

Symptoms

Most symptoms assoçiated with ulnar neuritis occur in the hand. These symptoms include:

- Intermittent or constant numbness and tingling in the ring finger and little finger, occurring most when the elbow bends.
- Difficulty with finger coordination and weakening of the grip. These symptoms are usually found in more severe cases.
- If the nerve is compressed for a long time or is very compressed, muscle wasting in the hand can occur. Once muscle wasting has occurred, the effects cannot be revered.

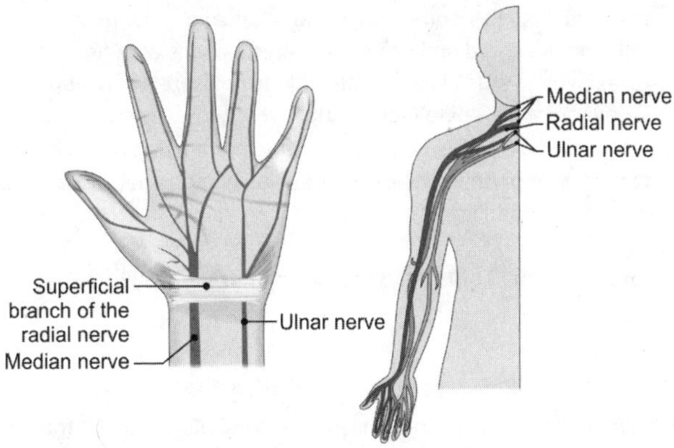

41. Glossopharyngeal nerve supplies which gland?

a. Parotid gland
b. Sweat gland
c. Thyroid gland
d. Sebaceous gland

Ans. a. Parotid gland

(Ref: Gray's Anatomy 41st edition, page 226)

- The glossopharyngeal nerve provides parasympathetic innervation to the parotid gland. These fibers originate in the inferior salivatory nucleus of CN IX. These fibers travel with the tympanic nerve to the middle ear. From the ear, the fibers continue as the lesser petrosal nerve, before synapsing at the otic ganglion.
- The fibers then hitchhike on the auriculotemporal nerve to the parotid gland, where they have a secretomotor effect.
- Remember—although the facial nerve splits into its five terminal branches in the parotid gland, it is the glossopharyngeal nerve that actually supplies the gland.

42. Defect seen due to failure of closure of rostral part of neural tube or cranial neuropore:

a. Anencephaly
b. Spina bifida
c. Osteogenesis
d. Cranium bifidum

Ans. a. Anencephaly

(Ref: Harrison's Principles of Internal Medicine 20th edition, vol 2, page 385)

- Failure of closure of the anterior neuropore during embryogenesis will lead to anencephaly, the failure of the brain and skull to develop. In less severe situations it may lead to different forms of encephalocele (i.e. cranium bifidum).
- There are three forms of cranium bifidum: (1) mengocele, (2) meningoencephalocele and (3) meningohydroencephalocele. In which respectively protrude the meninges, the meninges and brain tissue and lastly meninges, brain tissue and cranial ventricles.
- Failure of closure of the posterior neuropore (caudal neuropore) during embryogenesis will lead to spina bifida. This condition is always marked by a local lack of osteogenesis, or bone growth.
- The reason is that the correct differentiation and placement of underlying tissues (the spinal chord and spinal nerves and associated tissues) induce the osteogenesis, even small flaws in the underlying tissues can lead to a problem in the formation of the spine (vertebra).
- Occasionally spina bifida is accompanied by a protrusion of the meninges and cerebrospinal fluid (meningocele) or protrusion of meninges, cerebrospinal fluid and nerve tissue (meningomyelocele).

43. Cranial nerve carries parasympathetic fibers:

a. Vagus nerve
b. Optic nerve
c. Olfactory nerve
d. Accessory nerve

Ans. a. Vagus nerve *(Ref: Guyton and Hall 13th edition, page 439)*

- The only cranial nerves that transmit parasympathetic fibers are the oculomotor, facial, glossopharyngeal, and vagus nerves.
- Loss of function of the vagus nerve (X) will lead to a loss of parasympathetic innervation to a very large number of structures. Major effects of damage to the vagus nerve may include a rise in blood pressure and heart rate. Isolated dysfunction of only the vagus nerve is rare, but–if the lesion is located above the point at which the vagus first branches off–can be diagnosed by a hoarse voice, due to dysfunction of one of its branches, the recurrent laryngeal nerve.

44. Deep inguinal ring is found in which layer of anterior abdominal wall?

a. Transversalis fascia
b. Inferior gastric artery
c. Spermatic cord
d. Pubic symphysis

Ans. a. Transversalis fascia *(Ref: Gray's Anatomy 41st edition, page 449)*

There are two openings to the inguinal canal:

1. The deep or internal ring is located just above the midpoint of the inguinal ligament and lateral to the epigastric vessels. The deep ring is formed by the transversalis fascia which provides the posterior covering of the contents of the inguinal ring.

2. The superficial or external ring is the terminal end of the inguinal canal. It is located just superior to the pubic tubercle. The superficial ring has a triangular shape that is made by fibers of the external oblique muscle. These fibers continue to cover the inguinal contents as they descend into the scrotal area. Contiguous with the superficial ring are tendinous fibers (i.e. interligamentous fibers) which function to prevent the ring from enlarging.

45. First line of defense against tumor and viruses:

a. NK cells
b. Active hexose correlated compound
c. Granzymes
d. Hematopoiesis

Ans. a. NK cells

(Ref: Robbins Basic Pathology 10th edition, page 386)

- Natural killer (NK) cells serve as a crucial first line of defense against tumors and a diverse range of pathogens. Recognition of infection by NK cells is accomplished by the activation of receptors on the NK cell surface, which initiate NK cell effector functions.
- Many of the receptors and ligands involved in NK cell antimicrobial activity have been identified, and we are beginning to appreciate how they function during infection. In addition, NK cells are activated by cytokines (e.g. interleukin 12 and type I interferons), which are products of activated macrophages and dendritic cells.
- In response to these activating stimuli, NK cells secrete cytokines and chemokines and lyse target cells. Recent studies have focused on the mechanisms by which NK cells recognize and respond to viruses, parasites and bacteria, and on the unique role of NK cells in innate immunity to infection.

46. Acute graft rejection occurs within:

a. 1 year
b. 1 month
c. 2 years
d. 10 years

Ans. b. 1 month

(Ref: Bailey and Love's Short Practice of Surgery, 27th edition, page 532)

Acute Rejection

Developing with formation of cellular immunity, acute rejection occurs to some degree in all transplants, except between identical twins, unless immunosuppression is achieved (usually through drugs). Acute rejection begins as early as one week after transplant, the risk being highest in the first 3 months, though it can occur months to years later. Highly vascular tissues such as kidney or liver often host the earliest signs—particularly at endothelial cells lining blood vessels—though it eventually occurs in roughly 10 to 30% of liver transplants, and 10 to 20% of kidney transplants. A single episode of acute rejection can be recognized and promptly treated, usually preventing organ failure, but recurrent episodes lead to chronic rejection. It is believed that the process of acute rejection is mediated by the cell mediated pathway, specifically by mononuclear macrophages and T-lymphocytes. Histology of acute rejection is defined by dense lymphocytic cellular infiltrate as well as vasculitis of organ donor vessels.

Chronic Rejection

The term chronic rejection initially described long-term loss of function in transplanted organs via fibrosis of the transplanted tissue's blood vessels. This is now chronic allograft vasculopathy, however, leaving chronic rejection referring to rejection due to more patent aspects of immunity.

47. Type of cancer in Barrett's esophagus:

a. Basal cell carcinoma
b. Squamous cell carcinoma
c. Invasive ductal carcinoma
d. Adenocarcinoma

Ans. d. Adenocarcinoma *(Ref: Robbins Basic Pathology 10th edition, page 538)*

- Barrett's esophagus is a premalignant–not malignant–condition. It is malignant sequela, esophagogastric junctional adenocarcinoma, has a mortality rate of over 85%.
- The risk of developing esophageal adenocarcinoma in people who have Barrett's esophagus has been estimated to be 6–7 per 1,000 person-years, however a cohort study of 11,028 patients from Denmark published in 2011 showed an incidence of only 1.2 per 1,000 person-years (5.1 per 1,000 person-years in patients with dysplasia, 1.0 per 1,000 person-years in patients without dysplasia).
- The relative risk of esophageal adenocarcinoma is approximately 10 in those with Barrett's esophagus, compared to the general population. Most patients with esophageal carcinoma survive less than 1 year.

48. Type 2 hypersensitivity:

a. Pernicious anemia
b. Henoch–Schönlein purpura
c. Hashimoto's thyroiditis
d. Multiple sclerosis

Ans. a. Pernicious anemia *(Ref: Robbins Basic Pathology 10th edition, page 376)*

Type I/allergy/atopy (IgE)	Atopic eczema • Allergic urticaria • Allergic rhinitis (Hay fever) • Allergic asthma • Anaphylaxis • Food allergy – Common allergies include: Milk – Egg – Peanut – Tree nut – Seafood – Soy – Wheat • Penicillin allergy
Type II/ADCC • IgM • IgG	• Autoimmune hemolytic anemia • Immune thrombocytopenic purpura • Bullous pemphigoid • Pemphigus vulgaris • Rheumatic fever • Goodpasture syndrome • Guillain–Barré syndrome • Graves' disease • Myasthenia gravis Pernicious anemia

Contd...

Contd...

Type III (Immune complex)	• Henoch–Schönlein purpura • Hypersensitivity vasculitis • Reactive arthritis • Farmer's lung • Post-streptococcal glomerulonephritis • Serum sickness • Arthus reaction • Systemic lupus erythematosus • Subacute bacterial endocarditis Rheumatoid arthritis
Type IV Cell-mediated (T cells)	• Allergic contact dermatitis • Mantoux test • Diabetes mellitus type 1 • Hashimoto's thyroiditis • Multiple sclerosis • Coeliac disease • Giant-cell arteritis • Postorgasmic illness syndrome • Reactive arthritis • Transfusion-associated graft versus host disease

49. The earliest change in iron deficiency anemia:

a. Decreased serum iron
b. Decreased serum ferritin
c. Decreased TIBC
d. Decreased haemoglobin

Ans. b. Decreased serum ferritin

(Ref: Robbins Basic Pathology 10th edition, page 302)

Change in lab values in iron deficiency anemia	
Change	**Parameter**
↓	Ferritin, hemoglobin, mean corpuscular volume, mean corpuscular hemoglobin
↑	Total iron-binding capacity, transferrin, red blood cell distribution width

Iron-deficiency anemia is confirmed by tests that include serum ferritin, serum iron level, serum transferrin, and total iron binding capacity.

A low serum ferritin is most commonly found. However, serum ferritin can be elevated by any type of chronic inflammation and thus is not consistently decreased in iron-deficiency anemia.

Serum iron levels may be measured, but serum iron concentration is not as reliable as the measurement of both serum iron and serum iron-binding protein levels.

The percentage of iron saturation (or transferrin saturation index or percent) can be measured by dividing the level of serum iron by total iron binding capacity and is a value that can help to confirm the diagnosis of iron-deficiency anemia; however, other conditions must also be considered, including other types of anemia.

50. Which anemia shows low ESR?

a. Sickle cell anemia
b. Rheumatoid arthritis
c. Multiple myeloma
d. Waldenstrom's macroglobulinemia

Ans. a. Sickle cell anemia *(Ref: Robbins Basic Pathology 10th edition, page 302)*

The normal reference range for erythrocyte sedimentation rate (ESR) results is 1–13 mm/hr for males and 1–20 mm/hr for females. These values can also vary depending on the person's age. People with ESR results outside the standard range may have a medical condition.

Low levels

People with low ESR values may have:

- Sickle cell anemia, a condition that affects the shape of red blood cells
- Leukemia, a blood cell cancer
- A high red blood cell count
- Congestive heart failure
- Low levels of the protein fibrinogen in the blood
- Hyperviscosity, an increase in blood thickness
- A very high white blood cell count.

Moderately Elevated Results

A moderately elevated ESR may not always indicate a health condition.

However, it is possible that people whose ESR value is slightly high may have one of the following conditions:

- Rheumatoid arthritis
- Anemia, a reduced number of red blood cells
- Thyroid disease
- Kidney disease
- Red blood cell abnormalities, such as macrocytosis
- Some forms of cancer, such as lymphoma
- Tuberculosis, a type of lung infection
- A bone infection
- A heart infection
- A systemic infection.

Extremely Elevated Results

An extremely high ESR value, which is one above 100 mm/hr, may indicate one of these conditions:

- Multiple myeloma, a cancer of plasma cells
- Waldenstrom's macroglobulinemia, a white blood cell cancer
- Temporal arteritis or polymyalgia rheumatica
- Hypersensitivity vasculitis, a reaction to an allergen that results in blood vessel inflammation.

51. All of the following are derived from internal iliac lymph node *except*:

a. Ovaries
b. Rectum
c. Uterus
d. Bladder

Ans. a. Ovaries

(Ref: Gray's Anatomy 41st edition, page 302)

- The internal iliac lymph nodes surrounded the intestinal iliac artery and its branch (the hypogastric vessels), receive the lymphatics corresponding to the distribution of the branch of it.
- They receive lymphatics from all the pelvic viscera, from the deeper parts of the perineum, including the membranous and cavernous potions of the urethra, from the buttock and back of the thigh.
- It does not receive lymph from the ovary, testis or superior half ot the rectum.
- The gonads drain into the paraortic lymph nodes, while the superior half of the rectum drains to the pararectal lymph nodes.

52. All are true about anemia of chronic disease *except*:

a. High TIBC
B. High Ferritin
c. INC IL-6
d. Low TIBC

Ans. a. High TIBC

(Ref: Robbins Basic Pathology 10th edition, page 432)

While no single test is reliable to distinguish iron deficiency anemia from the anemia of chronic inflammation, there are sometimes some suggestive data:

- In anemia of chronic inflammation without iron deficiency, ferritin is normal or high, reflecting the fact that iron is sequestered within cells, and ferritin is being produced as an acute phase reactant. In iron deficiency anemia ferritin is low.
- Total iron-binding capacity (TIBC) is high in iron deficiency, reflecting production of more transferrin to increase iron binding; TIBC is low or normal in anemia of chronic inflammation.

53. Enzyme deficient in maple syrup urine disease:

a. Branched chain amino acid transaminase
b. Acyl CoA dehydrogenase
c. Alpha ketoacid decarboxylase
d. Isovaleryl CoA dehydrogenase

Ans. a. Branched chain amino acid transaminase

(Ref: Harpers Illustrated Biochemistry 31st edition, page 92)

- Maple syrup urine disease (MSUD) is an autosomal recessive metabolic disorder affecting branched-chain amino acids.
- It is one type of organic acidemia. The condition gets its name from the distinctive sweet odor of affected infants' urine, particularly prior to diagnosis, and during times of acute illness.

54. Primary compound found in fatty acid synthesis:

a. Acetyl CoA
b. Succinyl CoA
c. Malonyl-CoA
d. Acyl CoA

Ans. c. Malonyl-CoA *(Ref: Harpers Illustrated Biochemistry 31st edition, page 172)*

- Malonyl-CoA is formed by carboxylating acetyl-CoA using the enzyme acetyl-CoA carboxylase. One molecule of acetyl-CoA joins with a molecule of bicarbonate, requiring energy rendered from ATP.

- Malonyl-CoA is utilized in fatty acid biosynthesis by the enzyme malonyl coenzyme A : acyl carrier protein transacylase (MCAT). MCAT serves to transfer malonate from malonyl-CoA to the terminal thiol of holo-acyl carrier protein (ACP).

55. Key enzyme of gluconeogenesis *except*:

a. Glucose 6 phosphatase
b. Fructose 2,6 bisphosphatase
c. Pyruvate carboxylase
d. Phosphofructokinase

Ans. d. Phosphofructokinase

(Ref: Harpers Illustrated Biochemistry 31st edition, page 382)

Key steps and enzymes of gluconeogenesis

Substrate	Enzyme	Product
Pyruvate	*Pyruvate carboxylase* →	Oxaloacetate
Oxaloacetate	*PEP carboxykinase* →	PEP
Fructose- 1, 6-bisphosphatase	*Fructose- 1, 6-bisphosphatase* →	Fructose-6 phosphate
Glucose-6-phosphate	*Glucose-6-phosphatase* →	Glucose

Hexokinase/glucokinase, phosphofructokinase, and pyruvate kinase enzymes of glycolysis are replaced with glucose-6-phosphatase, fructose-1,6-bisphosphatase, and phosphoenolpyruvate (PEP) carboxykinase/pyruvate carboxylase.

56. Winging of scapula is due to paralysis of:

a. Serratus anterior muscle
b. Pectoralis major muscle
c. Rhomboidus major muscle
d. Lastissimus dorsi muscle

Ans. a. Serratus anterior muscle *(Ref: Gray's Anatomy 41st edition, page 433)*

- Winging of the scapula is divided into two categories, medial and lateral, according to the direction of winging.
- Medial winging is more common, being caused by serratus anterior paralysis.
- This is typically due to damage (i.e. lesions) of the long thoracic nerve.

57. Most abundant amino acid in collagen?

a. Glycine
b. Alanine
c. Arginine
d. Methionine

Ans. a. Glycine *(Ref: Harpers Illustrated Biochemistry 31st edition, page 629)*

- The most common motifs in the amino acid sequence of collagen are glycine-proline-X and glycine-X-hydroxyproline, where X is any amino acid other than glycine, proline or hydroxyproline.
- The average amino acid composition for fish and mammal skin is given.

58. NO is synthesized by:

a. Citrulline
b. Arginine
c. Alanine
d. Cysteine

Ans. b. Arginine

(Ref: Harpers Illustrated Biochemistry 31st edition, page 440)

- Nitric oxide synthases (NOSs) are a family of enzymes catalyzing the production of nitric oxide (NO) from L-arginine.
- Arginine, also known as l-arginine (symbol Arg or R), is an α-amino acid that is used in the biosynthesis of proteins.
- It is the precursor for the biosynthesis of NO. It is encoded by the codons CGU, CGC, CGA, CGG, AGA, and AGG.

59. Main LDL receptor is:

a. APO-A
b. APO-B-100
c. APOc-100
d. APO-100 and APO-E

Ans. b. APO-B-100 *(Ref: Harpers Illustrated Biochemistry 31st edition, page 55)*

- The low-density lipoprotein (LDL) receptor (LDL-R) is a mosaic protein of 839 amino acids (after removal of 21-amino acid signal peptide) that mediates the endocytosis of cholesterol-rich LDL.
- It is a cell-surface receptor that recognizes the apoprotein B100.

60. Which coenzyme is not a part of PDH?

a. NAD
b. FMN
c. FAD
d. CoA

Ans. b. FMN *(Ref: Harpers Illustrated Biochemistry 31st edition, page 201)*

The oxidation of pyruvate occurs in the mitochondria of the cell. The mitochondria is an organelle in the cell. It is considered the “powerhouse” of the cell. Pyruvate is transported there via pyruvate translocase. Pyruvate dehydrogenase is a multi-enzyme complex that uses three enzymes:

1. E1: Pyruvate dehydrogenase which uses thiamine pyrophosphate (TPP) as its prosthetic group.
2. E2: Dihydrolipoyl transacetylase which uses lipoamide and coenzyme A (also known as coASH) as its prosthetic groups.
3. E3: Dihydrolipoyl dehydrogenase which uses flavin adenine dinucleotide (FAD) and nicotinamide adenine dinucleotide (NAD^+) as its cofactors.

61. Adrenocorticol hormone is derived from:

a. Tyrosine
b. Tryptophan
c. Cholesterol
d. Cholecalciferol

Ans. c. Cholesterol *(Ref: Harpers Illustrated Biochemistry 31st edition, page 104)*

The synthesis of adrenocortical steroid hormones involves a chain of oxidation-reduction reactions catalyzed by a series of enzymes. Synthesis begins with a molecule of cholesterol.

Steroids are synthesized from cholesterol in their respective regions of the adrenal cortex.

62. Wernicke's encephalopathy is due to deficiency of:

a. VIT B1 b. VIT B2
c. VIT B6 d. VIT B12

Ans. a. VIT B1

(Ref: Robbins Basic Pathology 10th edition, page 331)

- Wernicke–Korsakoff syndrome (WKS), commonly known as wet brain, is the combined presence of Wernicke encephalopathy (WE) and alcoholic Korsakoff syndrome. Due to the close relationship between these two disorders, people with either are usually diagnosed with WKS as a single syndrome.
- The cause of the disorder is thiamine (vitamin B1) deficiency, which can cause a range of disorders including beriberi, Wernicke encephalopathy, and alcoholic Korsakoff syndrome.

63. Synthesis of type I collagen requires which vitamin?

a. VIT A b. VIT C
c. VIT D d. VIT K

Ans. b. VIT C

(Ref: Harpers Illustrated Biochemistry 31st edition, page 339)

Collagen keeps our skin firm and resilient, protecting it from wrinkling. The role of vitamin C in the production of collagen is to interact with amino acids within collagen cells. It adds hydrogen and oxygen to those amino acids, so that they may do their part in collagen production.

64. Catecholamines are synthesized from which amino acid?

a. Tryptophan b. Tyrosine
c. Lysine d. Threnine

Ans. b. Tyrosine

(Ref: Harpers Illustrated Biochemistry 31st edition, page 660)

- Catecholamines are derived from the amino acid tyrosine, which is derived from dietary sources as well as synthesis from phenylalanine.
- Catecholamines are water-soluble and are 50%-bound to plasma proteins in circulation.
- Tyrosine is created from phenylalanine by hydroxylation by the enzyme phenylalanine hydroxylase. Tyrosine is also ingested directly from dietary protein. Catecholamine-secreting cells use several reactions to convert tyrosine serially to L-DOPA and then to dopamine.

65. Resting membrane potential of RODS:

a. –30 mV b. –40 mV
c. –60 mV d. –70 mV

Ans. b. –40 mV *(Ref: Guyton and Hall 13th edition, page 202)*

- Unstimulated (in the dark), cyclic-nucleotide gated channels in the outer segment are open because cyclic GMP (cGMP) is bound to them.
- Hence, positively charged ions (namely sodium ions) enter the photoreceptor, depolarizing it to about −40 mV (resting potential in other nerve cells is usually −65 mV). This depolarization current is often known as dark current.

66. Dengue is caused by:

a. Anopheles
b. Culex
c. Aedes aegypti
d. Mansonoides

Ans. c. Aedes aegypti

(Ref: Park's Textbook of Preventive & Social Medicine 25th edition, page 204)

- Aedes aegypti, the yellow fever mosquito, is a mosquito that can spread dengue fever, chikungunya, Zika fever, Mayaro and yellow fever viruses, and other disease agents.
- The mosquito can be recognized by white markings on its legs and a marking in the form of a lyre on the upper surface of its thorax.

67. Most common type Hepatitis infection which leads to chronicity?

a. Hepatitis A
b. Hepatitis B
c. Hepatitis C
d. Hepatitis D

Ans. c. Hepatitis C

(Ref: Park's Textbook of Preventive & Social Medicine 25th edition, page 204)

- Hepatitis C virus (HCV) is a leading cause of chronic liver disease, cirrhosis, and hepatocellular carcinoma, as well as the most common indication for liver transplantation in many countries. Although the incidence of hepatitis C infection has dramatically decreased during the past decade, the worldwide reservoir of chronically infected persons is estimated at 170 million, or 3% of the global population. There is much controversy surrounding the natural history of hepatitis C infection.
- The rate of chronic HCV infection is affected by a person's age, gender, race, and viral immune response. Approximately 75–85% of HCV-infected persons will progress to chronic HCV infection, and are at risk for the development of extrahepatic manifestations, compensated and decompensated cirrhosis, and hepatocellular carcinoma (HCC).
- The rate of progression to cirrhosis is highly variable, and is influenced by several factors, including the amount of alcohol consumption, age of initial HCV infection, degree of inflammation and fibrosis on liver biopsy, HIV and HBV coinfection, and comorbid conditions.
- An estimated 10–15% of HCV-infected persons will advance to cirrhosis within the first 20 years. Persons with cirrhosis are at increased risk of developing HCC. An understanding of the natural history of hepatitis C is essential to effectively manage, treat, and counsel individuals with HCV infection.

68. Gastric emptying is maximum affected by:

a. Lipids
b. Amino acid
c. Carbohydrates
d. Fiber

Ans. a. Lipids *(Ref: Guyton and Hall 13th edition, page 438)*

- Its effect on solid meals is uncertain, and nothing is known of the effect on gastric emptying of fiber naturally present in food. This study therefore looked at gastric emptying of two different solid meals in eight healthy subjects and their blood glucose responses.
- The meals were exactly equivalent except for the total dietary fiber content (high fiber 20 g, low fiber 4 g of dietary fiber per 1,000 kcal) and supplied 870 kcal (700 kcal women), 47% of which was from carbohydrates, 36% from fats, and 17% from proteins.

69. Which is most internationally notifiable diseases under WHO?

a. Yellow fever
b. Polio
c. Diabetes
d. HTN

Ans. a. Yellow fever

(Ref: Park's Textbook of Preventive and Social Medicine 25th edition, page 392)

- The World Health Organization's International Health Regulations (WHO) 1969 require disease reporting to the organization in order to help with its global surveillance and advisory role. The current (1969) regulations are rather limited with a focus on reporting of three main diseases: cholera, yellow fever, and plague.
- The revised International Health Regulations 2005 broadens this scope and is no longer limited to the notification of specific diseases. While it does identify a number of specific diseases, it also defines a limited set of criteria to assist in deciding whether an event is notifiable to WHO.

70. Drug of choice for nasal carriers of MRSA is:

a. Linezolid
b. Mupirocin
c. Vancomycin
d. Teicoplanin

Ans. b. Mupirocin

(Ref: Essentials of Medical Pharmacology KDT 8th edition, page 371)

Mupirocin, sold under the brand name Bactroban among others, is a topical antibiotic useful against superficial skin infections such as impetigo or folliculitis. It may also be used to get rid of methicillin-resistant *S. aureus* (MRSA).

Vancomycin MIC > 2 μg/mL, an alternative to Vancomycin should be used. The approach is to treat with at least one agent to which VISA/VRSA is known to be susceptible by in vitro testing. The agents that are used include daptomycin, linezolid, telavancin, ceftaroline, quinupristin–dalfopristin.

Vancomycin (Note: For VRSA – DOC is daptomycin) (DOC for nasal carriers of MRSA – mupirocin).

71. Which of the following is a long acting insulin that never attains a peak concentration in plasma?

a. Insulin lispro
b. Insulin aspart
c. Insulin glargine
d. Insulin glulisine

Ans. c. Insulin glargine

(Ref: Essentials of Medical Pharmacology KDT 8th edition, page 203)

- Insulin glargine should not be mixed in the same syringe with any another insulin or solution because this will alter its pH and thus affect its absorption profile. Glargine has an onset of action of about 2 hours, and a duration of action of 20–24 hours.
- It may be given once daily at any time of day, or twice daily at higher doses (typically more than 50 units daily) to better maintain its relatively flat action profile.
- Its more consistent rate of absorption and lack of a significant peak action result in reduced nocturnal hypoglycemia when insulin glargine is used at bedtime compared with NPH insulin.

72. Which of the following drug cause Grey baby syndrome?

a. Tetracycline
b. Clindamycin
c. Vancomycin
d. Chloramphenicol

Ans. d. Chloramphenicol

(Ref: Essentials of Medical Pharmacology KDT 8th edition, page 402)

Gray baby syndrome (also termed Gray or Grey syndrome) is a rare but serious side effect that occurs in newborn infants (especially premature babies) following the accumulation of antibiotic chloramphenicol:

- The UDP-glucuronyl transferase enzyme system of infants, especially premature infants, is immature and incapable of metabolizing the excessive drug load.
- Insufficient renal excretion of the unconjugated drug.

73. Most common cause of blindness in India:

a. Cataract
b. Diabetes
c. Glaucoma
d. Trachoma

Ans. a. Cataract

(Ref: Comprehensive Ophthalmology by AK Khurana 7th edition, page 220)

The most common causes of blindness in 2010 were:

- Cataracts (51%)
- Glaucoma (8%)
- Age related macular degeneration (5%)
- Corneal opacification (4%)
- Childhood blindness (4%)
- Refractive errors (3%)
- Trachoma (3%)
- Diabetic retinopathy (1%)
- Undetermined (21%)[6]

About 90% of people who are visually impaired live in the developing world. Age-related macular degeneration, glaucoma, and diabetic retinopathy are the leading causes of blindness in the developed world.

74. Which diluent use to reconstitute BCG vaccine?

a. Normal saline
b. Ringer lactate
c. DNS
d. Distilled water

Ans. a. Normal saline

(Ref: Bailey & Love's Short Practice of Surgery, 27th edition, page 440)

Normal saline is recommended as a diluents to reconstituting the BCG vaccine, as distilled water may cause irritation. The reconstituted vaccine may be used up within 3 hours.

75. Zileuton is:

a. 5-lipoxygenase inhibitor
b. Cyclo-oxygenase inhibitor
c. Phospholipase inhibitor
d. Leukotriene receptor antagonist

Ans. a. 5-lipoxygenase inhibitor

(Ref: Essentials of Medical Pharmacology KDT 8th edition, page 330)

Zileuton is the only 5-lipoxygenase (5-LOX) inhibitor marketed as a treatment for asthma, and is often utilized as a selective tool to evaluate the role of 5-LOX and leukotrienes. The aim of this study was to investigate the effect of zileuton on prostaglandin (PG) production in vitro and in vivo.

76. Fulminant hepatitis is seen with which viral infection?

a. Hepatitis A
b. Hepatitis B
c. Hepatitis C
d. Hepatitis E

Ans. d. Hepatitis E

(Ref: Ananthanarayan and Paniker's Textbook of Microbiology 10th edition, page 394)

- Hepatitis E is inflammation of the liver caused by infection with the hepatitis E virus (HEV). One of five known human hepatitis viruses: A, B, C, D, and E, HEV is a positive-sense, single-stranded, nonenveloped, RNA icosahedral virus. HEV has mainly a fecal-oral transmission route
- Hepatitis E infection has a clinical course comparable to hepatitis A, but in pregnant women, the disease is more often severe and is associated with a clinical syndrome called fulminant liver failure.

77. Diagnosis of gout confirmed by which test?

a. Synovial fluid
b. X-ray
c. Blood test
d. NOTA

Ans. a. Synovial fluid

(Ref: Harrison's Principles of Internal Medicine 20th edition, vol 2, page 409)

- A definitive diagnosis of gout is based upon the identification of monosodium urate crystals in synovial fluid or a tophus.
- All synovial fluid samples obtained from undiagnosed inflamed joints by arthrocentesis should be examined for these crystals.
- Under polarized light microscopy, they have a needle-like morphology and strong negative birefringence.

78. Causative agent of Whipple's disease:

a. *Tropheryma whipplei*
b. Myxobacteria
c. *Haemophilus influenza*
d. Pseudomonas aeruginosa

Ans. a. Tropheryma whipplei

(Ref: Ananthanarayan and Paniker's Textbook of Microbiology 10th edition, page 320)

- Whipple's disease is a rare, systemic infectious disease caused by the bacterium *Tropheryma whipplei*.
- *Tropheryma whipplei*, formerly called Tropheryma whippelii, is a bacterium and the causative organism of Whipple's disease and, rarely, of endocarditis.
- While *T. whipplei* is categorized with the Gram-positive actinobacteria, the organism is commonly found to be Gram-positive or Gram-indeterminate when stained in the laboratory.
- Whipple himself probably observed the organisms as rod-shaped structures with silver stain in his original case.

79. Which antibody is suggestive of diagnosis of ulcerative colitis?

a. p-ANCA
b. c-ANCA
c. a.MA
d. a.NA

Ans. a. p-ANCA

(Ref: Harrison's Principles of Internal Medicine 20th Edition, Vol 1, Page 1269)

It is fairly specific, but not sensitive for ulcerative colitis, so is not useful as a sole diagnostic test. When measured together with anti-saccharomyces cerevisiae antibodies (ASCA), p-ANCA has been estimated to have a specificity of 97% and a sensitivity of 48% in differentiating patients with ulcerative colitis from normal controls.

80. Smoking is most common risk factor for which type of emphysema?

a. Panacinar
b. Centriacinar
c. Distal acinar
d. Irregular

Ans. b. Centriacinar *(Ref: Robbins Basic Pathology 10th edition, page 437)*

Three morphological types of emphysema:

1. Centriacinar begins in the respiratory bronchioles and spreads peripherally mainly in the upper half of the lungs and is usually associated with long-standing cigarette smoking.
2. Panacinar predominates in the lower half of the lungs and destroys the alveolar tissue and is associated with homozygous alpha-1 antitrypsin deficiency, a genetic disease.
3. Paraseptal emphysema preferentially localizes around the septae of the lungs or pleura, often associated with inflammatory processes, like prior lung infections.

81. Pappenheimer bodies are composed of:

a. Copper
b. Iron
c. Lead
d. Zinc

Ans. b. Iron *(Ref: Robbins Basic Pathology 10th edition, page 550)*

- Pappenheimer bodies are abnormal basophilic granules of iron found inside red blood cells on routine blood stain. They are a type of inclusion body composed of ferritin aggregates, or mitochondria or phagosomes containing aggregated ferritin.
- They appear as dense, blue-purple granules within the red blood cell and there are usually only one or two, located in the cell periphery.
- They stain on a Romanowsky stain because clumps of ribosomes are co-precipitated with the iron-containing organelles.

82. What is the genotype seen in Turner syndrome?

a. 45 + X0
b. 47,XXY
c. 47,XXX
d. 47,XX

Ans. a. 45 + X0 *(Ref: Robbins Basic Pathology 10th edition, page 760)*

- Turner syndrome (TS), also known 45,X, or 45,X0, is a genetic condition in which a female is partly or completely missing an X chromosome.
- Klinefelter syndrome (KS), also known as 47,XXY or XXY, is the set of symptoms that result from two or more X chromosomes in males. The primary features are infertility and small testicles.

- Triple X syndrome, also known as trisomy X and 47,XXX, is characterized by the presence of an extra X chromosome in each cell of a female.
- Down syndrome (DS or DNS), also known as trisomy 21, is a genetic disorder caused by the presence of all or part of a third copy of chromosome 21.

Abnormal karyotypes		
Karyotype	**Phenotype**	**Number of cases**
47,XY, + 21	Down syndrome	19
47,XX, + 21	Down syndrome	13
46,XY, t(13;21)	Down syndrome	1
46,XY, t(14;21)	Down syndrome	2
47,XY,+21/46,XY	Mosaic Down syndrome	1
47,XX, + 18	Edwards syndrome	3
47,XX, + 13	Patau syndrome	1
46,XY,del (5)(p14)	Mental retardation	1
46,XY,add (5)(q35.3)	Dysmorphic features	1
46,XY,del (10)(q26,2q36.3)	Mental retardation	1
46,XY,add (12)(p13.3)	Congenital anomalies	1
46,XY,add (15)(p26.3)	Mental retardation	1
46,XY,inv (9)(p11)	Dysmorphic features	1
46,XY,inv (9)(p11)	Mental retardation	1
47,XX, + mar/46,XX	Congenital malformations	1
47,XY, + mar/46,XY	Congenital malformations	1
45,X	Turner syndrome	2
45,X/46,XX	Mosaic turner syndrome	2
Total		53

83. Which of the following syndrome is related to obesity?

a. Cohen syndrome
b. Turner syndrome
c. Klinefelter syndrome
d. Mental retardation

Ans. a. Cohen syndrome

(Ref: Harrison's Principles of Internal Medicine 20th edition, vol 2, page 1192)

- Cohen syndrome (also known as Pepper syndrome or Cervenka syndrome) is a very rare autosomal recessive genetic disorder with varied expression, characterised by obesity, intellectual disability, distinct craniofacial abnormalities and potential ocular dysfunction.
- This syndrome is believed to be a gene mutation in chromosome 8 at locus 8q22 gene COH1. It has an autosomal recessive transmission with variable expression.There is evidence that this syndrome has a different mutation in the same gene as Mirhosseini–Holmes–Walton syndrome.

84. Calymmatobacterium is:

a. Gram-negative
b. Gram-positive
c. Acid fast
d. Non acid fast

Ans. a. Gram-negative

(Ref: Ananthanarayan and Paniker's Textbook of Microbiology 10th edition, page 502)

- *Klebsiella granulomatis* is Gram-negative, rod-shaped bacterium of the genus Klebsiella known to cause the sexually transmitted disease granuloma inguinale (or donovanosis).
- It was formerly called Calymmatobacterium granulomatis.

85. How much protein % of cow milk differ from human milk?

a. 2 times
b. 3 times
c. 4 times
d. 5 times

Ans. b. 3 times

(Ref: Harpers Illustrated Biochemistry 31st edition, page 402)

Comparing milks (per cup)			
Nutrient	**Human milk**	**Cow's milk (3.25% fat)**	**Goat's milk**
Calories (Kcal)	172	146	168
Water (g)	215	215	212
Protein (g)	2.5	7.9	8.7
Fat (g)	10.8	7.9	10.1
Saturated fat (g)	4.9	4.6	6.5
Monounsaturated fat (g)	4.1	2.0	2.7
Polyunsaturated fat (g)	1.2	0.5	0.4
Omega-3 fatty acids (mg)	128	183	97.6
Omega-6 fatty acids (mg)	920	293	266
Cholesterol (mg)	34.4	24.4	26.8
Carbohydrate (g)	17.0	11.0	10.9
Sugars (g)	17.0	11.0	10.9

86. Most common organ damage in Blunt trauma:

a. Spleen
b. Kidney
c. Heart
d. Liver

Ans. a. Spleen

(Ref: Bailey & Love's Short Practice of Surgery, 27th edition, page 403)

- Spleen is the most common cause of massive bleeding in blunt abdominal trauma to a solid organ. Spleen is the most commonly injured organ.
- The spleen is the second most commonly injured intra-abdominal organ in children.
- A laceration of the spleen may be associated with hematoma. Because of the spleen's ability to bleed profusely, a ruptured spleen can be life-threatening, resulting in shock.

- However, unlike the liver, penetrating trauma to the spleen, pancreas and kidneys do not present as much of an immediate threat of shock unless they lacerate a major blood vessel supplying the organs, such as the renal artery.
- Fractures of the left lower ribs are associated with spleen lacerations in 20% of cases.

87. Insulin which can be used in DKA?

a. Regular insulin
b. NPH insulin
c. Insulin lispro
d. Insulin glargine

Ans. a. Regular insulin

(Ref: Harrison's Principles of Internal Medicine 20th edition, vol 2, page 1187)

Treatment of DKA divided into four parts:

1. Correction of body's fluid
2. Administration of insulin
3. Correction of electrolyte abnormalities
4. Identification and treatment of precipitating events.

- 0.1 U/kg IV bolus of regular insulin, followed by 0.1 U/kg continuous infusion of regular insulin.
- If the serum glucose does not fall by mg/dL in the 1st hr, double the dose of infusion.
- When the serum glucose reach 200 mg/dL, reduce insulin infusion to 0.02–0.05 U/kg/hr.

88. KOH mount is done for:

a. Bacterial vaginosis
b. Candida
c. Syphilis
d. Chancroid

Ans. b. Candida

(Ref: Ananthanarayan and Paniker's Textbook of Microbiology 10th edition, page 300)

The KOH test for Candida albicans, also known as a potassium hydroxide preparation or KOH prep, is a quick, inexpensive fungal test to differentiate dermatophytes and Candida albicans symptoms from other skin disorders like psoriasis and eczema.

89. Incidence exposed/incidence non exposed:

a. Relative risk
b. Odds ratio
c. Forest plot
d. Hazard ratio

Ans. a. Relative risk

(Ref: Park's Textbook of Preventive and Social Medicine 25th edition, page 404)

- Risk ratio (RR) or relative risk is the ratio of the probability of an outcome in an exposed group to the probability of an outcome in an unexposed group.
- Risk ratio is used in the statistical analysis of the data of experimental, cohort and cross-sectional studies, to estimate the strength of the association between treatments or risk factors, and outcome.

90. Normal anion gap is maintained in which condition?

a. Renal tubular acidosis
b. Lactic acidosis
c. Ketoacidosis
d. Hypoalbuminemia

Ans. a. Renal tubular acidosis

(Ref: Harrison's Principles of Internal Medicine 20th Edition, Vol 2, Page 1482)

Low anion gap	Normal anion gap	High anion gap
• Hypoalbuminemia • Multiple myeloma	• Renal tubular acidosis • Addison's disease – Ammonium chloride • Acetazolamide • Ifosfamide • Hyperalimentation fluids (i.e. total parenteral nutrition) • Ketoacidosis	• Lactic acidosis • Ketoacidosis – Diabetic ketoacidosis – Alcohol abuse • *Toxins:* – Methanol – Ethylene glycol – Propylene glycol – Lactic acid – Uremia
		– Aspirin – Phenformin (no longer on market in U.S. since 1978 due to severe lactic acidosis, but still a problem globally. "Old metformin") – Iron – Isoniazid – Cyanide

91. Which IG increase in chronic disease?

a. IgG
b. IgM
c. IgA
d. IgD

Ans. a. IgG *(Ref: Harrison's Principles of Internal Medicine 20th Edition, Vol 2, Page 1458)*

The five subclasses of antibodies are:

1. Immunoglobulin A (IgA), which is found in high concentrations in the mucous membranes, particularly those lining the respiratory passages and gastrointestinal tract, as well as in saliva and tears.
2. Immunoglobulin G (IgG), the most abundant type of antibody, is found in all body fluids and protects against bacterial and viral infections, mainly seen in Chronic infection.
3. Immunoglobulin M (IgM), which is found mainly in the blood and lymph fluid, is the first antibody to be made by the body to fight a new infection.
4. Immunoglobulin E (IgE), which is associated mainly with allergic reactions (when the immune system overreacts to environmental antigens such as pollen or pet dander). It is found in the lungs, skin, and mucous membranes.
5. Immunoglobulin D (IgD), which exists in small amounts in the blood, is the least understood antibody.

92. hCG level in choriocarcinoma:

a. Inc
b. Dec
c. Constant
d. None

Ans. a. Inc *(Ref: DC Dutta's Textbook of Obstetrics 9th edition, Page 302)*

➢ Increased quantitative chorionic gonadotropin (hCG) (the "pregnancy hormone") levels
➢ Vaginal bleeding

- Shortness of breath
- Hemoptysis (coughing up blood)
- Chest pain
- Chest X-ray shows multiple infiltrates of various shapes in both lungs.

93. Cherry red discoloration is seen in which poisoning?

a. Nickel
b. Cyanide
c. Phosphorus
d. Carbon monoxide

Ans. d. Carbon monoxide

(Ref: Comprehensive Ophthalmology by AK Khurana 7th edition, page 203)

- One classic sign of carbon monoxide poisoning is more often seen in the dead rather than the living – people have been described as looking red-cheeked and healthy (*see* below).
- However, since this "cherry-red" appearance is more common in the dead, it is not considered a useful diagnostic sign in clinical medicine.
- In autopsy examinations, the ruddy appearance of carbon monoxide poisoning is notable because unembalmed dead persons are normally bluish and pale, whereas dead carbon-monoxide poisoned people may appear unusually lifelike in coloration.

94. A non hypertensive lady gets fluctuated BP during her pregnancy:

a. Pre-eclampsia
b. Chronic HTN
c. Gestational HTN
d. Eclampsia

Ans. c. Gestational HTN

(Ref: DC Dutta's Textbook of Obstetrics 9th edition, Page 201)

Hypertensive disease of pregnancy, also known as maternal hypertensive disorder, is a group of diseases that includes preeclampsia, eclampsia, gestational hypertension, and chronic hypertension.

Gestational Hypertension

Gestational hypertension is usually defined as having a blood pressure higher than 140/90 measured on two separate occasions, more than 6 hours apart, without the presence of protein in the urine and diagnosed after 20 weeks of gestation.

Pre-eclampsia

Pre-eclampsia is gestational hypertension plus proteinuria (>300 mg of protein in a 24-hour urine sample). Severe pre-eclampsia involves a blood pressure greater than 160/110, with additional medical signs and symptoms. HELLP syndrome is a type of pre-eclampsia. It is a combination of three medical conditions: hemolytic anemia, elevated liver enzymes and low platelet count.

Eclampsia

This is when tonic-clonic seizures appear in a pregnant woman with high blood pressure and proteinuria.

Pre-eclampsia and eclampsia are sometimes treated as components of a common syndrome.

95. Blood spillage on a ground? How to clean?

a. Propylene glycol
b. Formaldehyde
c. Ozone
d. Sodium hypochlorite

Ans. d. Sodium hypochlorite

(Ref: Harpers Illustrated Biochemistry 31st edition, page 302)

- Saturate the area again with sodium hypochlorite 0.5% (10,000 ppm available chlorine).
- This is a 1:10 dilution of 5.25% sodium hypochlorite bleach, which should be prepared daily.

96. Chronic malnutrition can be assessed by:

a. Height to age
b. Weight to age
c. Height to weight
d. Weight to height

Ans. a. Height to age

(Ref: Robbins Basic Pathology 10th edition, page 459)

- **Wasting:** Low weight-for-height is a sign of acute malnutrition : Indicator = prevalence of wasting
- **Stunting:** Low height-for-age is a sign of chronic malnutrition : Indicator = prevalence of stunting
- **Underweight:** Low weight-for-age is a sign of acute or chronic malnutrition or both : Indicator = prevalence of underweight
- Underweight is an internationally recognized public health indicator for monitoring nutritional status and health in populations.

97. Tissue bridging is seen in:

a. Stab wounds
b. Incised wounds
c. Lacerations
d. Abrasion

Ans. c. Lacerations

(Ref: Bailey & Love's Short Practice of Surgery, 27th edition, page 504)

- A laceration is defined as a tear in tissue caused by a shearing or crushing force. Therefore, a laceration is the result of a blunt-trauma mechanism.
- Because of the sharp-force mechanism of injury, incised wounds lack tissue bridging and often display very clean, sharp wound edges.

98. What is Quinsy?

a. Peritonsillar abscess
b. Retropharyngeal abscess
c. Sepsis
d. Michel de Montaigne

Ans. a. Peritonsillar abscess

(Ref: Dhingra's Diseases of ENT 7th edition, page 401)

- Peritonsillar abscess (PTA), also known as a quinsy, is pus due to an infection behind the tonsil.
- Symptoms include fever, throat pain, trouble opening the mouth, and a change to the voice.
- Pain is usually worse on one side. Complications may include blockage of the airway or aspiration pneumonitis.

99. A patient with HbsAg + HbeAg positive, what is the diagnosis?

a. Acute + infectivity
b. Acute + non-infective
c. Chronic + infectivity
d. Chronic + non-infective

Ans. a. Acute + infectivity *(Ref: Robbins Basic Pathology 10th edition, page 601)*

- The hepatitis B surface antigen (HBsAg) is most frequently used to screen for the presence of this infection.
- It is the first detectable viral antigen to appear during infection.
- Shortly after the appearance of the HBsAg, another antigen called hepatitis B e antigen (HBeAg) will appear. It's a sign of acute infectivity.

100. Which of the following receptor activated in hypercapnia?

a. Chemoreceptors
b. Cell surface receptor
c. Sensory receptor
d. Molecular sensor

Ans. a. Chemoreceptors *(Ref: Guyton and Hall 13th edition, page 300)*

- Hypercapnia normally triggers a reflex which increases breathing and access to oxygen (O_2), such as arousal and turning the head during sleep.
- A failure of this reflex can be fatal, for example as a contributory factor in sudden infant death syndrome.
- Hypercapnia can induce increased cardiac output, an elevation in arterial blood pressure (higher levels of carbon dioxide stimulate aortic and carotid chemoreceptors with afferents -CN IX and X- to medulla oblongata with following chrono- and inotropic effects), and a propensity toward cardiac arrhythmias. Hypercapnia may increase pulmonary capillary resistance.

101. Half-life of tritium is:

a. 6 hours
b. 3 days
c. 10 months
d. 12 years

Ans. d. 12 years *(Ref: Morgan and Mikhail's Clinical Anesthesiology, 6th edition, Page 192)*

Tritium is a radioactive isotope of the element hydrogen. Tritium is radioactive and has a half-life of about 12.5 years, which means that half of the radioactive atoms will decay naturally in that time.

102. Which is not done in papillary thyroid Ca in a pregnant female?

a. Radioactive exposure
b. Perform safe follow-up
c. Maintain optimal levels of maternal thyroxin
d. Balance of maternal calcium

Ans. a. Radioactive exposure

(Ref: Bailey & Love's Short Practice of Surgery, 27th edition, page 832)

Treatment and follow-up of thyroid cancer in pregnant women are the same as in non-pregnant patients except for the use of radioactive iodine. There are some differences in the management of the two most important histotypes: DTC (differentiated thyroid cancer: follicular and papillary cancer) and MTC (medullary thyroid cancer) just as for non-pregnant patients.

Pregnancy following thyroid cancer needs both maternal and foetal control.

The main problems are:

- To reach an adequate balance of maternal thyroid hormones that is absolutely required by the foetal central nervous system for normal maturation
- To maintain maternal levels of l-thyroxin to avoid possible recurrence or spread of disease
- To perform safe follow-up controls for the mother and to plan further therapy when needed.

103. Which of the following is marker of pheochromocytoma?

a. Vanillylmandelic acid (VMA) b. Fluorodopamine
c. Adrenomedullin d. Somatostatin

Ans. a. Vanillylmandelic acid (VMA)

(Ref: Robbins Basic Pathology 10th edition, page 174)

- Urinary VMA is elevated in patients with tumors that secrete catecholamines.
- These urinalysis tests are used to diagnose an adrenal gland tumor called pheochromocytoma, a tumor of catecholamine-secreting chromaffin cells.
- These tests may also be used to diagnose neuroblastomas, and to monitor treatment of these conditions.

104. All are example of nephrotic syndrome *except*:

a. Minimal change GN b. Focal segmented GN
c. Post streptococcal GN d. Membranous GN

Ans. c. Post streptococcal GN

(Ref: Robbins Basic Pathology 10th edition, page 523)

Nephrotic syndrome	Nephritic syndrome
• Primary causes • Minimal change glomerulonephritis • Focal segmental glomerulosclerosis • Membranous glomerulonephritis • Secondary causes • Systemic lupus erythematosus (SLE) • Hep B and C • HIV • Diabetes mellitus • Malignancy	• Post-streptococcal glomerulonephritis—appears weeks after upper respiratory tract infection (URTI) • IgA nephropathy—appears within a day or two after a URTI • Rapidly progressive glomerulonephritis (crescentic glomerulonephritis) • Goodpasture's syndrome—anti-GBM antibodies against basal membrane antigens • Vasculitic disorder—Wegener's granulomatosis, microscopic polyangiitis, churg strauss disease • Membranoproliferative glomerulonephritis—primary or secondary to SLE, Hepatitis B/C • Henoch-Schönlein purpura—systemic vasculitis—deposition of IgA in the skin and kidneys

105. A 40-year-male is presented to the emergency with dry gangrene on his legs? He was chronic smoker. His clinical scenarios describe:

a. Berger's disease b. Thromboangiitis obliterans
c. DVT d. Chronic venous insufficiency

Ans. b. Thromboangiitis obliterans

(Ref: Harrison's Principles of Internal Medicine 20th edition, vol 2, page 583)

- Thromboangiitis obliterans, also known as Buerger disease (English/bɜːrgər/, German/byrgər/), is a recurring progressive inflammation and thrombosis (clotting) of small and medium arteries and veins of the hands and feet.
- It is strongly associated with use of tobacco products, primarily from smoking.
- Chronic inflammation and thrombosis of arteries and veins of the hands and feet. The main symptom is pain in the affected areas, at rest and while walking (claudication).
- The impaired circulation increases sensitivity to cold. Peripheral pulses are diminished or absent. There are color changes in the extremities. The color may range from cyanotic blue to reddish blue.
- Skin becomes thin and shiny. Hair growth is reduced. Ulcerations and gangrene in the extremities are common complications, often resulting in the need for amputation of the involved extremity.

106. Which of the following is non-iodinated contrast?

a. Gadolinium
b. Visipaque
c. Iopamidol
d. Ditriazoate

Ans. a. Gadolinium

(Ref: The Basics and Fundamentals of Imaging 4th edition, page 20)

- Gadolinium has no known native biological role, but its compounds are used as research tools in biomedicine. Gd^{3+} compounds are components of MRI contrast agents.
- It is used in various ion channel electrophysiology experiments to block sodium leak channels and stretch activated ion channels.
- Gadolinium agents are useful for patients with renal impairment, in patients with severe renal failure requiring dialysis, there is a risk of a rare but serious illness called nephrogenic systemic fibrosis (NSF) or nephrogenic fibrosing dermopathy, that is linked to the use of MRI contrast agents containing gadolinium rest all other are iodinated contrast except gadolinium.

107. Rodent ulcer is seen in:

a. Squamous cell Ca
b. Basal cell Ca
c. Urinary bladder
d. Microaerophilic streptococci

Ans. b. Basal cell Ca

(Ref: Robbins Basic Pathology 10th edition, page 543)

- Rodent ulcer (also known as a "Jacob's ulcer") is a large skin lesion of nodular basal-cell carcinoma with central necrosis.
- Basal-cell carcinoma is a common skin cancer and occurs mainly in fair-skinned patients with a family history of this cancer.
- Sunlight is a factor in about two-thirds of these cancers; therefore, doctors recommend sunscreens with at least SPF 30.
- The use of a chemotherapeutic agent such as 5-fluorouracil or imiquimod can prevent development of skin cancer.

108. Which of the following disease is not included in vision 2020?

a. Refractive errors
b. Corneal blindness
c. Diabetic retinopathy
d. Trachoma

Ans. d. Trachoma

(Ref: Comprehensive Ophthalmology by AK Khurana 7th edition, page 392)

- **VISION 2020:** The Right to Sight was launched in 1999. It sought to promote: "A world in which nobody is needlessly visually impaired, where those with unavoidable vision loss can achieve their full potential."
- **The Global Initiative was set up to:** "Intensify and accelerate prevention of blindness activities so as to achieve the goal of eliminating avoidable blindness by 2020."
- **It sought to do this by:** "Focussing initially on certain diseases which are the main causes of blindness and for which proven cost effective interventions are available."
- The VISION 2020 Global Initiative has subsequently been complemented and avoidable blindness, but to include visual impairment—particularly that caused by uncorrected refractive error, refractive errors, childhood and corneal blindness, glaucoma and diabetic retinopathy.

109. Chest compression in adult is done at the rate of:

a. 50 compression per min
b. 100 compression per min
c. 150 compression per min
d. 200 compression per min

Ans. b. 100 compression per min

(Ref: Guyton and Hall 13th edition, page 293)

Chest Compressions

- The compression rate for adult cardiopulmonary resuscitation (CPR) is approximately 100 per minute (Class IIb).
- The compression-ventilation ratio for 1- and 2-rescuer CPR is 15 compressions to 2 ventilations when the victim's airway is unprotected (not intubated) (Class IIb).
- Chest compression—only CPR is recommended for use in dispatch-assisted CPR or when the rescuer is unwilling or unable to perform mouth-to-mouth rescue breathing (Class IIa).
- Audio prompts that guide action sequences and the timing of chest compressions and ventilations increase learning and retention of CPR skills and improve CPR performance (Class IIb).

110. A sensitive person, get affected easily and has difficulty in controlling anger and does not meet people? What is the personality defect?

a. Maniac
b. Borderline
c. Paranoid personality
d. Schizoid personality

Ans. b. Borderline

(Ref: Diagnostic and Statistical Manual of Mental Disorders 5th edition, page 129)

Borderline personality disorder (BPD), also known as emotionally unstable personality disorder (EUPD) pervasive pattern of unstable and intense interpersonal relationship, difficulty in controlling anger hence avoid meeting people.

111. What whould be the choice of initial treatment when a 65-year-old man with carotid artery stenosis develops severe depression and hypersomnia?

a. Doxepin
b. Phenelzine
c. Amitriptyline
d. Nortriptyline

Ans. d. Nortriptyline

(Ref: Harrison's Principles of Internal Medicine 20th edition, vol 2, page 832)

- Elderly patients are often sensitive to the hypotensive, sedative and anticholinergic effects of antidepressants.
- This patient is at special risk for hypotension because of his carotid artery stenosis.
- Nortriptyline is least likely to cause these side effects.

112. Sodium fluoride (NaF) inhibit which enzyme of glycolysis cycle?

a. Enolase
b. Hexokinase
c. Glucokinase
d. NOTA

Ans. a. Enolase

(Ref: Harpers Illustrated Biochemistry 31st edition, page 438)

- Fluoride acts primarily by inhibiting enolase in the glycolytic pathway. Fluoride strongly inhibits the enzyme in the presence of inorganic phosphate. The inhibitory species is the fluorophosphate ion, which when bound to magnesium forms a complex with enolase and inactivates the enzyme.
- Fluoride inhibits enolase, which is far downstream in the glycolytic pathway. Enzymes upstream of enolase remain active and continue to metabolize glucose until substrates are exhausted.

113. Which part of breast does progesterone act?

a. Ligaments
b. Lobules
c. Stroma
d. Ducts

Ans. d. Ducts

(Ref: Guyton and Hall 13th edition, page 726)

The main parts of the female breast are lobules (milk producing glands), ducts (milk passages that connect the lobules and the nipple), and stroma (fatty tissue and ligaments surrounding the ducts and lobules, blood vessels, and lymphatic vessels).

The complex physiology of breastfeeding includes a delicate balance of hormones. There are four hormones that help your breasts make milk: estrogen, progesterone, prolactin and oxytocin:

- Estrogen and progesterone prepare your breasts to make milk. These hormones are released by the placenta during pregnancy. They have two major roles. They increase the size and number of milk ducts in your breasts. They also keep your body from making large amounts of breast milk until after your baby is born.
- Prolactin helps your breasts make milk. After the birth of your baby, prolactin levels increase. Every time you breastfeed or pump, your body releases prolactin. With each release, your body makes and stores more milk in the breast alveoli.
- Oxytocin releases milk from your breasts. When your baby (or breast pump) begins to suck and draw your nipple into her mouth, this hormone is released.

114. Which of the following is seen in catatonia?

a. Cataplexy
b. Echolalia
c. Positivism
d. Disobedience

Ans. b. Echolalia

(Ref: Diagnostic and Statistical Manual of Mental Disorders 5th edition, page 182)

- Catatonia is a state of psycho-motor immobility and behavioral abnormality manifested by stupor. It was first described in 1874 by Karl Ludwig Kahlbaum, in German:
- Echolalia can be an indicator of communication disorders in autism, but is neither unique to, nor synonymous with syndromes.
- Echophenomena (particularly echolalia and echopraxia) were defining characteristics in the early descriptions of Tourette syndrome (TS).
- Echolalia also occurs in aphasia, schizophrenia, dementia, catatonia, epilepsy.

115. A long acting insulin, which does not attain peak concentration in plasma?

a. Humulin R
b. Glargine
c. Novolin R
d. Apidra

Ans. b. Glargine

(Ref: Essentials of Medical Pharmacology KDT 8th edition, page 928)

Rapid-acting: These include Apidra, Humalog, and Novolog. They have an onset in less than 15 minutes, peak in 30 to 90 minutes, and duration of 3 to 5 hours.

Regular (short-acting): These include Humulin R and Novolin R. They have an onset of a half an hour to 1 hour, a peak of two to four hours, and duration of 3 to 5 hours.

Long-acting insulin:

- Insulin glargine (Lantus), lasts up to 24 hours.
- Insulin detemir (Levemir), lasts 18 to 23 hours.
- Insulin glargine (Toujeo), lasts more than 24 hours.
- Insulin degludec (Tresiba), lasts up to 42 hours.
- Insulin glargine (Basaglar), lasts up to 24 hours.

116. Causing miscarriage without woman's consent comes under which IPC?

a. IPC 312
b. IPC 313
c. IPC 314
d. IPC 315

Ans. b. IPC 313

(Ref: Park's Textbook of Preventive & Social Medicine 25th edition, page 382)

Provisions under IPC

- Sec. 312–316 of IPC: Unlawful termination of pregnancy
- Sec. 312: Causing miscarriage
- Sec. 313: Causing miscarriage without consent of women
- Sec. 314: Death of a women by act done with intent to cause miscarriage
- Sec. 315: Act done with intent to prevent child being born alive or to cause it to die after birth
- Sec. 316-316: Causing death of quick unborn child by act amounting to culpable homicide

117. All of the following are feature of delirium *except*:

a. Sleep disturbance
b. Psychomotor disturbance
c. Sundowning
d. Rare cloudiness of consciousness

Ans. d. Rare cloudiness of consciousness

(Ref: Diagnostic and Statistical Manual of Mental Disorders 5th edition, page 218)

Delirium vs. Dementia vs. Depression			
Features	**Delirium**	**Dementia**	**Depression**
Onset	Acute (hours to days)	Insidious (months to years)	Acute or insidious (weeks to months)
Course	Fluctuating	Progressive	May be chronic
Duration	Hours to weeks	Months to years	Months to years
Consciousness	Altered	Usually clear	Clear
Attention	Impaired	Normal except in severe dementia	May be decreased
Psychomotor changes	Increased or decreased	Often normal	May be slowed in severe cases
Reversibility	Usually	Irreversible	Usually

118. A patient is on mechanical ventilation in ICU. Ventilator shows alarms for inc. in both peak and plateau pressure during inspiration. This indicates:

a. Obstruction of tracheal tube
b. Acute bronchospasm
c. Increase compliance of lungs
d. Decease in distensibility of lungs and chest wall

Ans. a. Obstruction of tracheal tube

(Ref: Guyton and Hall 13th edition, page 215)

Setting off of an alarm for peak inspiratory pressure during ventilation indicates an endotracheal tube kinking/obstruction.

Complications of intubation include:

- Damage to the vocal cords
- Bleeding
- Infection
- Tearing or puncturing of tissue in the chest cavity that can lead to lung collapse
- Injury to throat or trachea
- Tracheal tube obstruction by secretions, kinking
- Damage to dental work or injury to teeth
- Fluid buildup
- Aspiration.

119. Which of the following is not a tumor market for testicular carcinoma?

a. SP1
b. FSH
c. AFP
d. HCG

Ans. b. FSH *(Ref: Bailey & Love's Short Practice of Surgery, 27th edition, page 283)*

Head, neck	SCC	Nervous system	5-HIAA
Lungs	CEA SCC/NSE Cyfra 21–1	Thyroid	CEA Calcitonin Thyroglobulin
Liver	AFP	Esophagus	SCC
Bladder	CEA Cyfra 21–1 TPA	Breast	CEA CA 15–3 MCA Estrogen receptors Progesterone receptors
Colon, rectum	CEA CEA 19–9 CA 50	Stomach	CEA CA 72–4 CA50
Prostate	PSA PAP	Pancreas	CA 19–9 Elastase
Testis	β-hCG AFP SP-1	Ovary	CEA CA 125 AFP β-hCCG
Blood	β2-microglobulin	Cervix	SCC

120. Which of the following cancer arise from Barrett's esophagus?

a. Squamous cell carcinoma
b. Adenocarcinoma
c. Insulinoma
d. Pheochromocytoma

Ans. b. Adenocarcinoma

(Ref: Bailey & Love's Short Practice of Surgery, 27th edition, page 283)

- Barrett's esophagus is a condition in which there is an abnormal (metaplastic) change in the mucosal cells lining the lower portion of the esophagus, from normal stratified squamous epithelium to simple columnar epithelium with interspersed goblet cells that are normally present only in the stomach, small intestine, and large intestine.
- This change is considered to be a premalignant condition because it is associated with a high incidence of further transition to esophageal adenocarcinoma, an often-deadly cancer.

121. Hoffmann degradation is seen in metabolism of:

a. NO
b. Pancuronium
c. Atracurium
d. Vecuronium

Ans. c. Atracurium *(Ref: Guyton and Hall 13th edition, page 762)*

- Atracurium, a nondepolarizing muscle relaxant, is eliminated through several pathways, including Hofmann elimination (spontaneous degradation in plasma and tissue at normal body pH and temperature) and ester hydrolysis (catalysis by nonspecific esterase)

- **Hofmann elimination provided precisely this basis:** It is a chemical process in which a suitably activated quaternary ammonium compound can be degraded by the mildly alkaline conditions present at physiological pH and temperature.
- In effect, Hofmann elimination is a retro-Michael addition chemical process. It is important to note here that the physiological process of Hofmann elimination differs from the non-physiological Hofmann *degradation* process.
- **Hofmann degradation process:** The latter is a chemical reaction in which a quaternary ammonium hydroxide solid salt is heated to 100°C, or an aqueous solution of the salt is boiled.

122. Exercise intolerance with muscle cramp is seen in which glycogen storage disease?

a. Cori's disease
b. Hers disease
c. Pompe's disease
d. McArdle's disease

Ans. d. McArdle's disease

(Ref: Harpers Illustrated Biochemistry 31st edition, page 39)

Type	Defective enzyme	Organ affected	Glycogen in the affected organ	Clinical features
I. Von Gierke	Glucose 6-phosphatase or transport system	Liver and kidney	Increased amount; normal structure	Massive enlargement of the liver. Failure to thrive. Severe hypoglycemia, ketosis, hyperuricemia, hyperlipidemia
II. Pompe	α-1,4-Glucosidase (lysosomal)	All organs	Massive increase in amount; normal structure	Cardiorespiratory failure causes death, usually before age 2
III. Cori	Amylo-1,6-glucosidase (debranching enzyme)	Muscle and liver	Increased amount; short outer branches	Like type I, but milder course
IV. Andersen	Branching enzyme (α-1,4 → α-1,6)	Liver and spleen	Normal amount; very long outer branches	Progressive cirrhosis of the liver. Liver failure causes death, usually before age 2
V. McArdle	Phosphorylase	Muscle	Moderately increased amount; noral structure	Limited ability to perform strenuous exercise because of painful muscle cramps. Otherwise patient is normal and well developed
VI. Hers	Phosphorylase	Liver	Increased amount	Like type I, but milder course
VII.	Phosphofructo-kinase	Muscle	Increased amount; normal structure	Like type V
VIII.	Phosphorylase kinase	Liver	Increased amount; normal structure	Mild liver enlargement. Mild hypoglycemia

Note: Types I through VII are inherited as autosomal recessives. Type VIII is sex linked.

Type	Affected tissue	Enzyme defect	Clinical features	Tissue needed for diagnosis*	Outcome
i. Von Gierke's disease	Liver intestine, kidney	Glucose-6-Phosphatase	Hepatomegaly, hypoglycemia, stunted growth, obesity, hypotonia	Liver	If patients survive initial hypoglycemia, prognosis is good; hyperuricemia is a late complication
ii. Pompe's disease	Liver, muscle, heart	Lysosomal α-glucosidase	Heart failure, cardiomyopathy	Leukocytes, liver, muscle	Death in first 6 months; juvenile and adult variants seen
iii. Forbes' disease	Liver, muscle (abnormal glycogen structure)	Amylo-1, 6-glucosidase	Like Type 1	Leukocytes, liver, muscle	Good prognosis
iv. Andersen disease	Liver (abnormal glycogen structure)	1,4-α-glucan branching enzyme	Failure to thrive, hepatomegaly, cirrhosis and its complications	Leukocytes, liver, muscle	Death in first 3 years
v. McArdle disease	Muscle only	Phosphorylase	Muscle cramps and myoglobinuria after exercise (in adults)	Muscle	Normal lifespan; exercise must be avoided

* Tissue obtained is used for the biochemical assay of the enzyme

123. McNaughten's rule related to?

a. Insanity
b. Infancy
c. Intoxications
d. Consent

Ans. a. Insanity

(Ref: Diagnostic and Statistical Manual of Mental Disorders 5th edition, page 216)

Insanity or mental abnormality (Section-84)	
Conditions of insanity	**Kinds of unsound mind**
Wrong must be done by a unsound mind • Person is incapable to understand – Nature of crime – Act is against law • This incapability is due to unsoundness of mind	1. Idiot 2. Lunatic 3. Non compos mentis 4. Disease of mind
Important Case-laws	
• Mc Naughten's case • Someswar Ghora vs. State of Assam—1981 Crl. J. NOC 51 Gauhati—Legal insanity has to be proved before the court, not medical insanity • Ratan Lal vs State of MP—AIR 1971SC778—Setting fire to one's own house & cloths without any reason is considered insanity • Babu Dev vs State of Pepsu (Panjab)—AIR 1956 SC488—Insanity as a result of smoking ganja or heavy intoxication making a person thoroughly insane is valid defence under section 84	

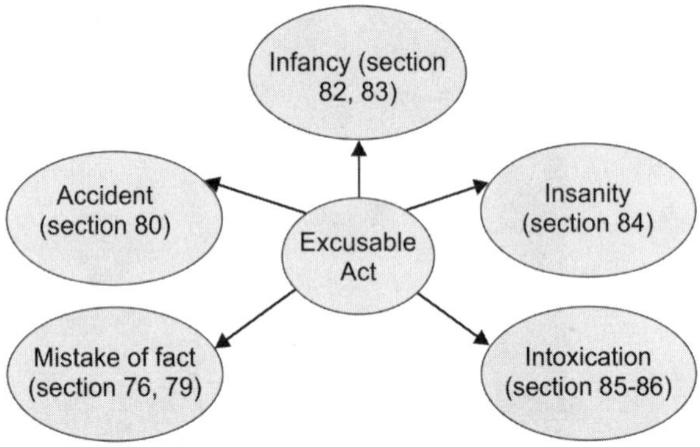

124. Malignant hyperthermia is caused by:

a. Ryanodine receptor
b. Nicotinic receptor
c. Muscarinic receptor
d. NMDA receptor

Ans. a. Ryanodine receptor

(Ref: Guyton and Hall 13th edition, page 328)

- Malignant hyperthermia's inheritance is autosomal dominant with variable penetrance. The defect is typically located on the long arm of chromosome 19 (19q13.2) involving the Ryanodine receptor.
- More than 25 different mutations in this gene are linked with malignant hyperthermia.

- These mutations tend to cluster in one of three domains within the protein, designated MH1-3. MH1 and MH2 are located in the N-terminus of the protein, which interacts with L-type calcium channels and Ca^{2+}.
- MH3 is located in the transmembrane forming C-terminus.

125. Which of the following is uncoupler of oxidative phosphorylation?

a. Antimycin A
b. 2, 4-Dinitrophenol
c. Oligomycin
d. Rotenone

Ans. b. 2, 4-Dinitrophenol

(Ref: Harpers Illustrated Biochemistry 31st edition, page 402)

Compounds	Use	Site of action	Effect on oxidative phosphorylation
Cyanide, Carbon monoxide, Azide, Hydrogen sulfide	Poisons	Complex IV	Inhibit the electron transport chain by binding more strongly than oxygen to the Fe–Cu center in cytochrome c oxidase, preventing the reduction of oxygen.
Oligomycin	Antibiotic	Complex V	Inhibits ATP synthase by blocking the flow of protons through the Fo subunit.
CCCP 2,4-Dinitrophenol	Poisons, weight-loss	Inner membrane	Ionophores that disrupt the proton gradient by carrying protons across a membrane. This ionophore uncouples proton pumping from ATP synthesis because it carries protons across the inner mitochondrial membrane.
Rotenone	Pesticide	Complex I	Prevents the transfer of electrons from complex I to ubiquinone by blocking the ubiquinone-binding site.
Malonate and oxaloacetate	Poisons	Complex II	Competitive inhibitors of succinate dehydrogenase (complex II).
Antimycin A	Piscicide	Complex III	Binds to the Qi site of cytochrome C reductase, thereby inhibiting the oxidation of ubiquinol.

126. Vitamin which help in iron absorption:

a. VIT A
b. VIT B
c. VIT C
d. VIT D

Ans. c. VIT C

(Ref: Harpers Illustrated Biochemistry 31st edition, page 299)

- Vitamin C has been shown to enhance iron absorption.
- It captures non-heme iron and stores it in a form that is more easily absorbed by your body.
- Foods high in vitamin C include citrus fruits, dark green leafy vegetables, bell peppers, melons and strawberries.

127. Most common site of Fordyces spot:

a. Lips
b. Axilla
c. Groin
d. Below tongue

Ans. a. Lips

(Ref: Robbins Basic Pathology 10th edition, page 932)

- Fordyce spots are whitish-yellow bumps that can occur on the edge of your lips or inside your cheeks.
- Less often, they can appear on your penis or scrotum if you're male or your labia if you're female.
- The spots, also called Fordyce granules or Fordyce glands, are enlarged oil glands.

128. In intestine glucose is Cotransported by:

a. SGLT1
b. SGLT2
c. SGLT3
d. SGLT4

Ans. a. SGLT1

(Ref: Harpers Illustrated Biochemistry 31st edition, page 324)

- Sodium-dependent glucose cotransporters (or sodium-glucose linked transporter, SGLT) are a family of glucose transporter found in the intestinal mucosa (enterocytes) of the small intestine (SGLT1) .
- The proximal tubule of the nephron (SGLT2 in PCT and SGLT1 in PST). They contribute to renal glucose reabsorption.
- In the kidneys, 100% of the filtered glucose in the glomerulus has to be reabsorbed along the nephron (98% in PCT, via SGLT2).

129. Farmer's lung is caused by:

a. Immediate hypersensitivity
b. Antibody mediated
c. Immune complexes
d. Cell-mediated

Ans. c. Immune complexes

(Ref: Robbins Basic Pathology 10th edition, page 649)

- Farmer's lung (not to be confused with silo-filler's disease) is a hypersensitivity pneumonitis induced by the inhalation of biologic dusts coming from hay dust or mold spores or any other agricultural products.
- It results in a type III hypersensitivity inflammatory response and can progress to become a chronic condition which is considered potentially dangerous.

130. Moth eaten alopecia is caused by:

a. Primary syphilis
b. Secondary syphilis
c. Tertiary syphilis
d. Early relapsing syphilis

Ans. b. Secondary syphilis

(Ref: Robbins Basic Pathology 10th edition, page 140)

- The frequency of hair loss in secondary syphilis ranges from 2.9% to 7%. The precise pathogenesis is unknown. The hair loss can be moth-eaten, diffuse or both.

- The "moth-eaten" pattern is the most common type and is considered to be a pathognomonic manifestation of secondary syphilis.The alopecia, which is nonscarring, can occasionally affect hair-bearing areas other than the scalp.
- The biopsy sample can be noninflammatory or show changes indistinguishable from alopecia areata *T. pallidum* is usually not seen with silver staining.
- The alopecia usually resolves within three months of appropriate treatment for syphilis.

131. Narrowest part of larynx in children:

a. Subglottis b. Glottis
c. Arytenoids cartilage d. Aryepiglottic folds

Ans. a. Subglottis *(Ref: Gray's Anatomy 41st edition, page 491)*

- The narrowest part of the adult airway is the vocal cords, but, in children, the narrowest part is the cricoid cartilage located in the subglottic area of the larynx.
- The subglottis or subglottic region is the lower portion of the larynx, extending from just beneath the vocal cords down to the top of the trachea.
- The structures in the subglottis are implicated in the regulation of the temperature of the breath.
- Narrowing of the subglottis is known as subglottic stenosis and may require a tracheotomy to correct.

132. A Confused patient was brought to emergency, opens the eye with painful stimulation and extends the arm on unilateral side on needle prick, what is his GCS score?

a. 7/15 b. 8/15
c. 9/15 d. 10/15

Ans. b. 8/15

(Ref: Bailey and Love's Short Practice of Surgery, 27th edition, page 382)

Glasgow Coma Scale

Behavior	Response	Score
Eye opening response	Spontaneously To speech To pain No response	4 3 2 1
Best verbal response	Oriented to time, place, and person Confused Inappropriate words Incomprehensible sounds No response	5 4 3 2 1
Best motor response	Obeys commands Moves to localized pain Flexion withdrawal from pain Abnormal flexion (decorticate) Abnormal extension (decerebrate) No response	6 5 4 3 2 1
Total score:	*Best response* *Comatose client* *Totally unresponsive*	15 8 or less 3

133. Which type of Anemia is seen in rheumatoid arthritis?

a. Hemolytic anemias
b. Hereditary spherocytosis
c. Polycythemia
d. Normocytic normochromic anemia

Ans. d. Normocytic normochromic anemia

(Ref: Harrison's Principles of Internal Medicine 20th Edition, Vol 2,Page 832)

A normochromic normocytic anemia is a common finding in patients suffering from RA with the patient's haemoglobin being mildly decreased with levels greater than 10 g/dL usually seen unless there has been chronic bleeding from vasculitis of the stomach, kidney and so on.

134. Which of the following are features of Inverse Retinitis pigmentosa?

a. X-linked
b. Bony spicule on fovea
c. Bony spicule on para fovea
d. Progressive choroid degeneration

Ans. a. X-linked

(Ref: Harrison's Principles of Internal Medicine 20th edition, vol 2, page 832)

- Retinitis pigmentosa (RP) is one of the most common forms of inherited retinal degeneration.
- There are multiple genes that, when mutated, can cause the retinitis pigmentosa phenotype.
- Inheritance patterns of RP have been identified as autosomal dominant, autosomal recessive, X-linked, and maternally (mitochondrially) acquired, and are dependent on the specific RP gene mutations present in the parental generation.
- In 1989, a mutation of the gene for rhodopsin, a pigment that plays an essential part in the visual transduction cascade enabling vision in low-light conditions, was identified.

135. Maximum content of VIT A is seen in:

a. Amla
b. Guava
c. Halibut liver oil
d. Lemon

Ans. c. Halibut liver oil

(Ref: Harpers Illustrated Biochemistry 31st edition, page 264)

Halibut liver oil:

- A supplementation high in Vitamin A with the benefits of Fish oil.
- Essential Fatty Acids (EFA) help prevent the formation of Triglycerides in the blood, stopping the blood from clotting which can help prevent heart disease and heart attacks.

136. Nasopharyngeal carcinoma causes deafness by:

a. CNX involvement
b. CNV involvement
c. A + B
d. Eustachian tube block

Ans. d. Eustachian tube block

(Ref: Dhingra's Diseases of ENT 7th edition, Page 325)

- Fluid accumulation is the most common cause of conductive hearing loss in the middle ear, especially in children.
- Major causes are ear infections or conditions that block the eustachian tube, such as allergies or tumors.

- Blocking of the eustachian tube leads to decreased pressure in the middle ear relative to the external ear, and this causes decreased motion of both the ossicles and the tympanic membrane.

Clinical Features

- **Severe Headache:** Indicates skull base erosion
- **Trotter's triad:**
  - **Conductive deafness:** Eustachian tube block
  - **+I/L temporo-parietal neuralgia:** Trigeminal damage
  - **+I/L palatal paralysis:** Vagus damage
- **Distant metastasis:** To bone, lung and liver

137. A 30-year-old patient presents with pain in right hypochondrium for 5 days with soft and tender liver and intercostal tenderness. He complains of catch in breath on inspiration and has a non-productive cough. On examination the lung fields clear, patient looks pale and emaciated. What is the probable diagnosis?

a. Amoebic liver abscess b. Pyogenic liver abscess
c. Hydatid cyst d. Hepatic adenoma

Ans. a. Amoebic liver abscess

(Ref: Harrison's Principles of Internal Medicine 20th edition, vol 1, Page 428)

Amoebic Liver Abscess

Symptoms

- Pain right hypochondrium referred to right shoulder
- Pyrexia (100.4 F)
- Profuse sweating and rigors
- Loss of weight
- Earthy complexion

Signs

- Pallor
- Tenderness and rigidity in right hypochondrium
- Palpable liver
- Intercostal tenderness
- Basal lung signs

138. Jack in a box is seen in:

a. Aphakia b. Cataract
c. Squint d. Pseudophakia

Ans. a. Aphakia

(Ref: Comprehensive Ophthalmology by AK khurana 7th edition, page 300)

- **Jack-in-the-box Phenomenon:** The presence of the above scotoma leads to another interesting phenomenon seen in Aphakia. If an interesting object appears in the periphery of the patients visual field, it appears blurred (because the light is passing from the side of the spectacle frame).
- The person tends to move his head towards the object in order to see it clearly. But as he turns the head the object comes to lie in the area of scotoma and thus disappears.

- As he turns his head further so that the object comes to lie in front of the spectacle in the visible area and so reappears again clear and sharp. This sudden disappears and sharp.

139. Which of the following is abductor of vocal cord?

a. Posterior cricoarytenoid
b. Cricothyroid muscle
c. Oblique arytenoid muscles
d. Transverse arytenoid muscle

Ans. a. Posterior cricoarytenoid

(Ref: Gray's Anatomy 41st edition, page 402)

The intrinsic laryngeal muscles are responsible for controlling sound production.

- Cricothyroid muscle lengthen and tense the vocal folds.
- Posterior cricoarytenoid muscles abduct and externally rotate the arytenoid cartilages, resulting in abducted vocal folds.
- Lateral cricoarytenoid muscles adduct and internally rotate the arytenoid cartilages, increase medial compression.
- Transverse arytenoid muscle adduct the arytenoid cartilages, resulting in adducted vocal folds.
- Oblique arytenoid muscles narrow the laryngeal inlet by constricting the distance between the arytenoid cartilages.
- Thyroarytenoid muscles—sphincter of vestibule, narrowing the laryngeal inlet, shortening the vocal folds, and lowering voice pitch. The internal thyroarytenoid is the portion of the thyroarytenoid that vibrates to produce sound.

140. A 50-year-old female, presented with redness, painful, sudden loss of vision. She also claims about seeing colored haloes. Diagnosis?

a. Keratitis
b. Retinal detachment
c. Acute congestive glaucoma
d. Angular conjunctivitis

Ans. c. Acute congestive glaucoma

(Ref: Comprehensive Ophthalmology by AK khurana 7th edition, page 235)

Acute congestive glaucoma usually presents with sudden painful loss of vision associated with colored haloes. ACG more commonly seen in middle to elderly females.

D/dx of color haloes:

- ACG
- Cataract
- Mucopurulent conjunctivitis (Not in angular)

RD presents with sudden painless loss of vision associated with flashes of light.

141. Most common affected site in Charcot's joints:

a. Foot
b. Hand
c. Chest
d. Back

Ans. a. Foot *(Ref: Rockwood and Green's Fractures in Adults 8th edition, page 388)*

Neuropathic arthropathy (or neuropathic osteoarthropathy), also known as Charcot joint (often Charcot foot) after the first to describe it, Jean-Martin Charcot, refers to progressive degeneration of a weight bearing joint, a process marked by bony destruction, bone resorption, and eventual deformity due to loss of sensation. Onset is usually insidious.

142. Diabetic nephropathy is characteristic by which nodule?

a. Toxic nodules
b. Kimmelstiel–Wilson nodules
c. Multibacterial nodular
d. Single bacterial nodule

Ans. b. Kimmelstiel–Wilson nodules

(Ref: Harrison's Principles of Internal Medicine 20th edition, vol 2, page 603)

Kimmelstiel–Wilson nodule

- Damage to the glomerular basement membrane allows proteins in the blood to leak through, leading to proteinuria.
- Deposition of abnormally large amounts of mesangial matrix causes periodic acid-Schiff positive nodules called Kimmelstiel–Wilson nodules.

143. Loss of migration of neural crest cells causes:

a. Achalasia
b. Hirschprung disease
c. Intestinal neuronal dysplasia
d. Ileus

Ans. b. Hirschprung disease

(Ref: Harrison's Principles of Internal Medicine 20th edition, vol 1, page 1046)

- During normal prenatal development, cells from the neural crest migrate into the large intestine (colon) to form the networks of nerves called the myenteric plexus (Auerbach plexus) (between the smooth muscle layers of the gastrointestinal tract wall).
- The submucosal plexus (Meissner plexus) (within the submucosa of the gastrointestinal tract wall).
- In Hirschsprung disease, the migration is not complete and part of the colon lacks these nerve bodies that regulate the activity of the colon.
- The affected segment of the colon cannot relax and pass stool through the colon, creating an obstruction.

144. Tolosa-Hunt syndrome involves:

a. Orbital floor
b. Orbital apex
c. Orbital roof
d. Orbital space

Ans. b. Orbital apex *(Ref: Dhingra's Diseases of ENT 7th edition, page 543)*

- Orbital apex syndrome, is a collection of cranial nerve deficits associated with a mass lesion near the apex of the orbit of the eye.
- This syndrome is a separate entity from Rochon–Duvigneaud syndrome, which occurs due to a lesion immediately anterior to the orbital apex. Most commonly optic nerve is involved.
- Tolosa-Hunt syndrome (THS) is a rare disorder characterized by severe and unilateral headaches with orbital pain, along with weakness and paralysis (ophthalmoplegia) of certain eye muscles (extraocular palsies).

145. A child had Chinese fried rice after 9 hours of consumption got diarrhea, which microorganism is responsible for this?

a. B. mycoides
b. B. pseudomycoides
c. B. weihenstephanensis
d. Bacillus cereus

Ans. d. Bacillus cereus

(Ref: Ananthanarayan and Paniker's Textbook of Microbiology 10th edition, page 552)

- Bacillus cereus is a gram-positive, rod-shaped, facultatively anaerobic, motile, beta-hemolytic, spore forming bacterium commonly found in soil and food.
- The bacteria is classically contracted from fried rice dishes that have been sitting at room temperature for hours.
- Cereus bacteria are facultative anaerobes, and like other members of the genus Bacillus, can produce protective endospores. Its virulence factors include cereolysin and phospholipase C.

146. Which of the following is WHO obesity index?

a. Broca index
b. Ponderal index
c. Quetelet index
d. Corpulence index

Ans. c. Quetelet index

(Ref: Park's Textbook of Preventive and Social Medicine 25th edition, page 834)

- Body mass index (BMI) old name Quetelet index is a value derived from the mass (weight) and height of a person.
- The BMI is defined as the body mass divided by the square of the body height, and is universally expressed in units of kg/m^2, resulting from mass in kilograms and height in metres.
- The Corpulence Index (CI) or Ponderal Index (PI) is a measure of leanness (corpulence) of a person.

147. Roth spots are seen in:

a. Infective endocarditis
b. Libman-Sacks endocarditis
c. NBTE
d. Hypertension retinopathy

Ans. a. Infective endocarditis *(Ref: Robbins Basic Pathology 10th edition, page 117)*

Roth spots, also known as Litten spots or the Litten sign, are non-specific red spots with white or pale centres, seen on the retina and although traditionally associated with infective endocarditis, can occur in a number of other conditions including hypertension, diabetes, Collagen vascular disease, extreme hypoxia, leukemia and HIV.

148. Which of the following is determining factor for severity of TOF?

a. ASD
b. RVH
c. Pulmonary stenosis
d. Overriding of aorta

Ans. c. Pulmonary stenosis *(Ref: Robbins Basic Pathology 10th edition, page 305)*

"Tetralogy" denotes four parts, here implying the syndrome's four anatomic defects.

- Pulmonary stenosis, narrowing of the exit from the right ventricle
- A ventricular septal defect, a hole between the two ventricles
- Right ventricular hypertrophy, thickening of the right ventricular muscle
- An overriding aorta, which allows blood from both ventricles to enter the aorta

The pulmonic stenosis is the major cause of the malformations, with the other associated malformations acting as compensatory mechanisms to the pulmonic stenosis. The degree of stenosis varies between individuals with TOF, and is the primary determinant of symptoms and severity. This malformation is infrequently described as subpulmonary stenosis or subpulmonary obstruction.

149. All seen with tumor lysis syndrome *except*:

a. Lactic acidosis
b. Hyperkalemia
c. Hyperuricemia
d. Hypercalcemia

Ans. d. Hypercalcemia

(Ref: Harrison's Principles of Internal Medicine 20th edition, vol 2, page 1284)

Tumor lysis syndrome is characterized by:

- High blood potassium (hyperkalemia)
- High blood phosphate (hyperphosphatemia)
- Low blood calcium (hypocalcemia)
- High blood uric acid (hyperuricemia)
- Higher than normal levels of blood urea nitrogen (BUN)
- Nitrogen-containing compounds (azotemia).

150. What is the treatment of Anderson-Gustilo classification grade 3B?

a. Intramedullary nailing
b. Intramedullary wiring
c. Close reduction
d. K wire

Ans. b. Intramedullary wiring

(Ref: Rockwood and Green's Fractures in Adults 8th edition, page 227)

- For open fractures like 3B intramedullary nails are preferred over K wires.
- Open fracture with extensive soft-tissue loss and periosteal stripping and bone damage.
- Usually associated with massive contamination. Will often need further soft-tissue coverage procedure (i.e. free or rotational flap).

151. Most common tumor of anterior mediastinum:

a. Branchial cyst
b. Branchial fistula
c. Thymoma
d. Parasitic cyst

Ans. c. Thymoma

(Ref: Bailey and Love's Short Practice of Surgery, 27th edition, page 362)

Thymoma:

- Most common primary anterior mediastinal tumor (20%) in adults but rarely seen in children. It can be classified as lymphocytic, epithelial, or spindle cell histologies, but the clinical significance of these classifications is controversial.
- Tonofibrils seen under electron microscopy can differentiate thymoma from other tumors such as carcinoid, Hodgkin's, and seminoma.
- The most common mediastinal masses are neurogenic tumors (20% of mediastinal tumors), usually found in the posterior mediastinum, followed by thymoma (15–20%) located in the anterior mediastinum.
- Lung cancer typically spreads to the lymph nodes in the mediastinum.

152. Most specific marker of MI:

a. Troponin test
b. Creatine Kinase (CK-MB) test
c. Lactate dehydrogenase (LDH)
d. Myoglobin (Mb)

Ans. a. Troponin test

(Ref: Harrison's Principles of Internal Medicine 20th edition, vol 2, page 364)

Troponin test: The most sensitive and specific test for myocardial damage. Because it has increased specificity compared with CK-MB, troponin is a superior marker for myocardial injury.

Creatine Kinase (CK-MB) test: It is relatively specific when skeletal muscle damage is not present.

LDH is not as specific as troponin whereas Mb have low specificity for myocardial infarction.

153. Kienböck disease is avascular necrosis of:

a. Scaphoid
b. Trapezoid
c. Lunate
d. Trapezium

Ans. c. Lunate *(Ref: Robbins Basic Pathology 10th edition, page 543)*

- Kienböck's disease is a disorder of the wrist. It is named for Dr. Robert Kienböck, a radiologist in Vienna, Austria who described osteomalacia of the lunate in 1910.
- It is breakdown of the lunate bone, a carpal bone in the wrist that articulates with the radius in the forearm
- Specifically, Kienböck's disease is another name for avascular necrosis (death and fracture of bone tissue due to interruption of blood supply) with fragmentation and collapse of the lunate.

154. Which cells release histamine?

a. Mast cell
b. Granulocyte
c. Mesangial cell
d. Endothelial cell

Ans. a. Mast cell *(Ref: Robbins Basic Pathology 10th edition, page 639)*

- Most histamine in the body is generated in granules in mast cells and in white blood cells (leukocytes) called basophils.
- Mast cells are especially numerous at sites of potential injury—the nose, mouth, and feet, internal body surfaces, and blood vessels.
- Non-mast cell histamine is found in several tissues, including the brain, where it functions as a neurotransmitter.

155. Most common defect in Down syndrome:

a. Ventricular septal defect
b. Secundum atrial septal
c. Tetralogy of Fallot
d. Endocardial cushion defect

Ans. a. Ventricular septal defect

(Ref: Robbins Basic Pathology 10th edition, page 742)

Down syndrome

The most common lesions were endocardial cushion defect (43%), ventricular septal defect (32%), secundum atrial septal defect (10%), tetralogy of Fallot (6%), and isolated patent ductus arteriosus (4%).

156. Most common site for metastasis in brain?

a. Liver
b. Lung
c. Kidney
d. Heart

Ans. b. Lung *(Ref: Robbins Basic Pathology 10th edition, page 852)*

The most common sources of brain metastases:

- Lung cancer, 48%
- Breast cancer, 15%
- Genitourinary tract cancers, 11%
- Osteosarcoma, 10%
- Melanoma, 9%
- Head and neck cancer, 6%
- Neuroblastoma, 5%
- Gastrointestinal cancers, especially colorectal and pancreatic carcinoma, 3%
- Lymphoma, 1%.

Lung cancer and melanoma are most likely to present with multiple metastasis, whereas breast, colon, and renal cancers are more likely to present with a single metastasis.

157. Osgood-Schlatter disease involves:

a. Tibial tuberosity b. Femoral condyle
c. Lateral malleolus d. Medial malleolus

Ans. a. Tibial tuberosity

(Ref: Rockwood and Green's Fractures in Adults 8th edition, page 231)

- Osgood-Schlatter disease (OSD) is a condition in which the patellar tendon insertion on the tibial tuberosity becomes inflamed.
- It is a well-known condition in late childhood characterized by pain and a bony prominence over the tibial tuberosity.
- The pain is usually exacerbated by physical activities like running, jumping, and climbing stairs.

158. Earliest finding in diabetic nephropathy:

a. Microalbuminuria b. Hyperglycemia
c. Increased blood pressure levels d. Genetic predisposition

Ans. a. Microalbuminuria

(Ref: Harrison's Principles of Internal Medicine 20th edition, vol 2, page 1432)

The first sign of diabetic kidney disease (nephropathy) is protein or albumin in the urine (microalbuminuria). If you have albumin in the urine and you are diabetic, you likely have diabetic nephropathy.

- Diabetic nephropathy is rare in adolescents and unusual in those who have been diagnosed for less than five years. However, microalbuminuria (incipient nephropathy) and even renal histological changes can be found a relatively short while after diagnosis in some diabetics.
- It is not clear what determines the rate of progression from incipient to overt nephropathy but hypertension, glomerular hyperfiltration, hypercholesterolemia, and poor glycemic control have been implicated.

159. Seat belt injury is commonly seen with:

a. Weakness b. Respiratory difficulty
c. Mesenteric tearing d. None

Ans. c. Mesenteric tearing

(Ref: Review of Forensic Medicine and Toxicology, 4th edition, page 132)

- Injury to abdominal viscera has been attributed to compression between the belt and the vertebral column, and the intestinal ischemia is primarily due to mesenteric tears.
- Mesenteric tears usually occur due to the shearing force applied on the mesentery, which happens while the movable intestines continue moving with the same speed of the car, although the car is decelerated by the act of the brakes (described in physics as the inertia).
- These tears can be so trivial that a frank intestinal ischemia would not be apparent immediately.

160. PHC covers population in plane area:

a. 20,000
b. 30,000
c. 40,000
d. 5,000

Ans. b. 30,000

(Ref: Park's Textbook of Preventive and Social Medicine 25th edition, page 973)

	Subcenter	PHC	CHC
Level of care	Primary	Primary	Secondary
Population norms			
Plains	5000	30,000	1,20,000
Hilly/tribal areas	3000	20,000	80,000
Staff	3	15	30
Maintenance	Central govt.	State govt.	State govt.
Rural area covered	21 sq. Km	140 sq. Km	770 sq. Km
Radial distance	2.6	6.6	15.6
Average number of villages covered	4	29	158

161. Image of iceberg phenomenon with value of 12 cases mentioned above the surface, 20 at the surface, 50 beneath the surface. Which disease has following pattern?

a. TB
b. Measles
c. Rabies
d. Tetanus

Ans. a. TB *(Ref: Park's Textbook of Preventive and Social Medicine 25th edition, page 635)*

- Iceberg phenomenon can be compared to a disease in community.
- **Floating tip of iceberg (Visible portion):** Clinical cases that physician seen in community. It can be detected by diagnostic test.
- **Submerged part (hidden portion):** are the latent, undiagnosed cases and carriers. It is detected by screening by an epidemiologist.
- **Iceberg phenomenon is not shown by:** Rabies – Tetanus – measles – rubella Whereas seen with TB.

162. Epidemic dropsy caused by which toxin?

a. Ergot alkaloids
b. Diphtheria toxin
c. Yohimbine
d. Sanguinarine argemone oil

Ans. d. Sanguinarine argemone oil

(Ref: Ananthanarayan and Paniker's Textbook of Microbiology 10th edition, page 452)

- Epidemic dropsy is a form of edema of extremities due to poisoning by Argemone mexicana (Mexican prickly poppy).
- Epidemic dropsy is a clinical state resulting from use of edible oils adulterated with Argemone mexicana seed oil.
- Sanguinarine and dihydrosanguinarine are two major toxic alkaloids of argemone oil, which cause widespread capillary dilatation, proliferation and increased capillary permeability.
- When mustard oil is adulterated deliberately (as in most cases) or accidentally with argemone oil, proteinuria (specifically loss of albumin) occurs, with a resultant edema as would occur in nephrotic syndrome.

163. Folic acid supplement required during pregnancy:

a. 400 mg
b. 500 mg
c. 600 mg
d. 700 mg

Ans. a. 400 mg

(Ref: Park's Textbook of Preventive and Social Medicine 25th edition, page 833)

- Folic acid is a pregnancy superhero! Taking a prenatal vitamin with the recommended 400 micrograms (mcg) of folic acid before and during pregnancy can help prevent birth defects of your baby's brain and spinal cord.
- Take it every day and go ahead and have a bowl of fortified cereal, too.
- It may be taken by mouth or by injection. The recommended adult daily intake of folate in the US is 400 micrograms from foods or dietary supplements.
- Folate in the form of folic acid is used to treat anemia caused by folate deficiency.

164. Which of the following hypoxia is seen with inadequate utilization of oxygen?

a. Hypoxic hypoxia
b. Hypemic hypoxia
c. Stagnant hypoxia
d. Histotoxic hypoxia

Ans. d. Histotoxic hypoxia *(Ref: Guyton and Hall 13th edition, page 742)*

Hypoxia, in medicine, condition of the body in which the tissues are starved of oxygen. In its extreme form, where oxygen is entirely absent, the condition is called anoxia.

There are four types of hypoxia

1. The hypoxemic type, in which the oxygen pressure in the blood going to the tissues is too low to saturate the hemoglobin.
2. The anemic type, in which the amount of functional hemoglobin is too small, and hence the capacity of the blood to carry oxygen is too low.
3. The stagnant type, in which the blood is or may be normal but the flow of blood to the tissues is reduced or unevenly distributed.
4. The histotoxic type, in which the tissue cells are poisoned and are therefore unable to make proper use of oxygen. Diseases of the blood, the heart and circulation, and the lungs may all produce some form of hypoxia.

165. Which genetic condition leads to spontaneous abortion?

a. Trisomy 13
b. Trisomy 16
c. Trisomy 18
d. Trisomy 21

Ans. b. Trisomy 16 *(Ref: DC Dutta's Textbook of Obstetrics 9th edition, page 634)*

- Miscarriage, also known as spontaneous abortion and pregnancy loss, is the natural death of an embryo or fetus before it is able to survive independently
- Trisomy 16 is a chromosomal abnormality in which there are 3 copies of chromosome 16 rather than two. It is the most common trisomy leading to miscarriage and the second most common chromosomal cause of it, closely following X-chromosome monosomy.
- About 6% of miscarriages have trisomy 16. Those mostly occur between 8 to 15 weeks after the last menstrual period.
- It is not possible for a child to be born alive with an extra copy of this chromosome present in all cells (full trisomy 16). It is possible, however, for a child to be born alive with the mosaic form.

166. From 1970–1995, 500 people were monitored. Exposed to smoking 400, Non-exposed 100. Out of 400 exposed 50 developed the lung cancer and out of 100 non-exposed 5 developed the lung cancer. Calculate the relative risk.

a. 1.2 b. 2.5
c. 1.5 d. 3.5

Ans. b. 2.5 *(Ref: Park's Textbook of Preventive and Social Medicine 25th edition, page 1029)*

Relative risk (RR) or risk ratio is the ratio of the probability of an outcome in an exposed group to the probability of an outcome in an unexposed group.

	Disease (+)	Disease (–)	Total
Exposed	50	350	400
Non-exposed	5	95	100

Putting the value in formula

= 50/400 % 5/100

= 50/400 × 5/100

RR = 2.5

167. Titres seen in rheumatic fever:

a. ASO b. VDRL
c. Wassermann test d. mCHIP

Ans. a. ASO *(Ref: Harrison's Principles of Internal Medicine 20th edition, vol 2, page 1326)*

- According to revised Jones criteria, the diagnosis of rheumatic fever can be made when two of the major criteria, or one major criterion plus two minor criteria, are present along with evidence of streptococcal infection: elevated or rising antistreptolysin O titre or DNAase.
- Exceptions are chorea and indolent carditis, each of which by itself can indicate rheumatic fever.
- Antistreptolysin O antibodies will be raised after infection with streptococci. Levels greater than 200 units per millilitre are considered significant (although cut off levels will vary between laboratory undertaking the test).
- Measurement can be useful diagnostically if recent infection with streptococci is known to be important in etiology. Diseases include:

- Rheumatic fever
- Post-streptococcal glomerulonephritis
- Scarlet fever
- Erysipelas

168. Killian's dehiscence occurs:

a. 1 bands of inferior constrictor
b. 2 bands of inferior constrictor
c. 1 bands of exterior constrictor
d. 2 bands of exterior constrictor

Ans. b. 2 bands of inferior constrictor

(Ref: Gray's Anatomy 41st edition, page 735)

- Killian's dehiscence (also known as Killian's triangle) is a triangular area in the wall of the pharynx between the two bands of the cricopharyngeus of the inferior constrictor of the pharynx (also *see* Pharyngeal pouch). It can be seen as a locus minoris resistentiae.
- Similar triangular area between circular fibers of cricopharyngeus and longitudinal fibers of esophagus is Lamier's triangle or Lamier-Hackermann's area. It represents a potentially weak spot where a pharyngoesophageal diverticulum (Zenker's diverticulum) is more likely to occur.

169. A 26-year-old patient presents with a history suggestive of TB. On examination he has pleural effusion. All of the following parameters will be used for analysis of pleural fluid *except*:

a. Gene XPERT
b. LDH
c. Albumin
d. ADA

Ans. c. Albumin *(Ref: Robbins Basic Pathology 10th edition, page 534)*

- Pleural effusion in TB could be a presentation of primary TB due to subpleural location of Gohn's focus or can present as extra pulmonary TB.
- Gene Xpert. The Gene Xpert is a new test for tuberculosis. It can find out if a person is infected with TB, and also if the TB bacterium of the person has resistance to one of the common TB drugs, rifampicin.
- LDH criteria also concern with pleural effusion
- Adenosine deaminase has 90% sensitivity and 92% specificity for determining the tubercular nature of fluid whereas Albumin values in serum and ascitis fluid are evaluated in patient of ascites not pleural effusion.

170. Umbilical artery carries:

a. Deoxygenated blood from the fetus to the placenta
b. Oxygenated blood from the fetus to the placenta
c. Deoxygenated blood from the placenta to the fetus
d. Oxygenated blood from the placenta to the fetus

Ans. a. Deoxygenated blood from the fetus to the placenta

(Ref: Guyton and Hall 13th edition, page 46)

- The umbilical artery (latin: arteria umbilicalis) is a branch of the anterior division of the internal iliac artery that functions only in the time of the placental blood circulation.
- The umbilical artery passes along the anterior wall of the abdominal cavity to the umbilical ring, it passes further in the umbilical cord to the placenta.

- After birth the umbilical artery obliterates and its distal part becomes the medial umbilical ligament, but the proximal part of the umbilical artery gives rise to the superior vesical arteries.
- The umbilical arteries supply deoxygenated blood from the fetus to the placenta. After birth, the superior vesical arteries from the umbilical artery supply the urinary bladder.

171. According to WHO Adolescent age is:

a. <1 year　　b. <19 years
c. >19 years　　d. >65 years

Ans. b. <19 years

(Ref: Park's Textbook of Preventive and Social Medicine 25th edition, page 763)

- Adolescence is transitional phase of growth and development between childhood and adulthood. The World Health Organization (WHO) defines an adolescent as any person between ages 10 and 19.
- This age range falls within WHO's definition of young people, which refers to individuals between ages 10 and 24.

172. A 35-year-old patients shows abnormal schilling test. Antibiotics were given for 5 days which results in normalization of schilling test. What is the diagnosis of patient?

a. Bacterial overgrowth syndrome　　b. Chronic pancreatitis
c. Atrophic gastritis　　d. Ileocecal TB

Ans. a. Bacterial overgrowth syndrome

(Ref: Harrison's Principles of Internal Medicine 20th edition, Vol 1, page 458)

- Schilling test helps in determine the etiology of VIT B12 deficiency
- Bacterial overgrowth syndrome occurs due to growth of large intestinal microbiota flora like bacteroides to multiply in small intestine.
- Hence after a course of antibiotics when the flora will die, normal B12 absorption can take place and Schilling's test will become normal.

173. Transport media for salmonella:

a. Buffered glycerol saline　　b. Normal saline
c. Hypertonic saline　　d. Quarter-normal saline

Ans. a. Buffered glycerol saline

(Ref: Ananthanarayan and Paniker's Textbook of Microbiology 10th edition, page 637)

Maintain viability of enteric pathogens while transporting stool specimens to the laboratory with Thermo Scientific™ Buffered Glycerol Saline. Collect, transport and preserve clinical specimens with a transport medium especially suited for Salmonella and Shigella species.

174. Most common clinical feature seen in prolactinoma next to galactorrhea:

a. Impotence　　b. Hypogonadism
c. Gynecomastia　　d. Amenorrhea

Ans. d. Amenorrhea

(Ref: Harrison's Principles of Internal Medicine 20th edition, vol 1, page 732)

- Amenorrhea (female patients)
- Galactorrhea (female patients)
- Infertility
- Decreased libido
- Impotence (male patients)
- Osteoporosis
- Delayed puberty (adolescents)
- Mass effect
- Headaches
- Visual acuity & field impairment
- Cranial nerve palsies
- Hypothalamic impairment hydrocephalus
- Hypopituitarism
- Pituitary apoplexy

175. Normal sperm concentration according to WHO:

a. 5 million/mL
b. 7 million/mL
c. 10 million/mL
d. 15 million/mL

Ans. d. 15 million/mL

(Ref: Park's Textbook of Preventive and Social Medicine 25th edition, page 473)

A normal sperm count ranges from 15 million sperm to more than 200 million sperm per milliliter (mL) of semen according to the WHO in 2010.

Anything less than 15 million sperm per milliliter, or 39 million sperm per ejaculate, is considered low. A low sperm count is often referred to as oligospermia.

A high, or above average, sperm count is over 200 million sperm per millimeter.

You can determine your sperm count through a semen analysis. You can get the analysis done at your doctor's office, a fertility clinic, or with an at-home test.

- **Aspermia:** Absence of semen
- **Azoospermia:** Absence of sperm
- **Hypospermia:** Low semen volume
- **Hyperspermia:** High semen volume
- **Oligozoospermia:** Very low sperm count
- **Asthenozoospermia:** Poor sperm motility
- **Teratozoospermia:** Sperm carry more morphological defects than usual
- **Necrozoospermia:** All sperm in the ejaculate are dead
- **Leucospermia:** A high level of white blood cells in semens.

176. Lucio phenomenon is seen in:

a. Lepromatous leprosy
b. Histoid leprosy
c. Leonine leprosy
d. Tuberculoid leprosy

Ans. a. Lepromatous leprosy

(Ref: Harrison's Principles of Internal Medicine 20th edition, vol 1, page 930)

- Lucio's phenomenon is an unusual reaction seen almost exclusively in patients from the Caribbean and Mexico with diffuse, lepromatous leprosy, especially in untreated cases
- It is characterized by recurrent crops of large, sharply demarcated, ulcerative lesions, affecting mainly the lower extremities, but may generalize and become fatal as a result of secondary bacteria infection and sepsis.

177. How much is the sodium concentration in ORS as per WHO?

a. 75 mmol/L
b. 65 mmol/L
c. 25 mmol/L
d. 35 mmol/L

Ans. a. 75 mmol/L

(Ref: Park's Textbook of Preventive and Social Medicine 25th edition, page 738)

Reduced osmolarity ORS	Grams/litre	Reduced osmolarity ORS	mmol/litre
Sodium chloride	2.6	Sodium	75
Glucose, anhydrous	13.5	Chloride	65
Potassium chloride	1.5	Glucose, anhydrous	75
Trisodium citrate, dihydrate	2.9	Potassium	20
		Citrate	10
		Total osmolarity	245

178. Average weight in pregnancy:

a. 10 kg
b. 12 kg
c. 16 kg
d. 18 kg

Ans. b. 12 kg *(Ref: DC Dutta's Textbook of Obstetrics 9th edition, page 534)*

Pre-pregnancy or early pregnancy (less than 10 weeks) BMI (kg/m^2)	Total weight gain range
Underweight (<18.5)	12.5 kg–18 kg
Healthy weight (18.5–24.9)	11.5 kg–16 kg
Overweight (25.0–29.9)	7 kg–11.5 kg
Obese (≥ 30.0)	5 kg–9 kg

179. A 12-year-old girl irritability, dry mouth and slow skin pinch. Next step of management:

a. Ringer lactate
b. ORS
c. Hydrational fluids
d. Plain water

Ans. a. Ringer lactate

(Ref: Bailey and Love's Short Practice of Surgery, 27th edition, page 475)

- For infants under one year of age, WHO recommends giving, within the first hour, 30 milliliters of Ringer's lactate solution for each kilogram of body weight, and then, within the next five hours, 70 milliliters of Ringer's lactate per kilogram of body weight.
- For children over one year and for adults, WHO recommends, within the first half hour, 30 milliliters of Ringer's lactate per kilogram of body weight, and then, within the next two-and-a-half hours, 70 milliliters per kilogram. For example, if a child weighs fifteen kilograms (who is obviously over one year of age), he or she should receive 450 mL of Ringer's Lactate Solution within the first half hour, and then 1,050 mL of Ringer's lactate within the next two-and-a-half hours.

180. Vaccines given post-splenectomy give protection from diseases caused by:

a. *S. pneumoniae*
b. *Haemophilus Influenzae*
c. *Neisseria meningitidis*
d. All of the above

Ans. d. All of the above

(Ref: Ananthanarayan and Paniker's Textbook of Microbiology 10th edition, page 524)

Recommendations

- **Level 1**
  - None
- **Level 2**
  - Non-elective splenectomy patients should be vaccinated on or after postoperative day 14.
  - Asplenic patients should be revaccinated at the appropriate time interval for each vaccine.
- **Level 3**
  - Elective splenectomy patients should be vaccinated at least 14 days prior to the operation.
  - Asplenic or immunocompromised patients (with an intact, but nonfunctional spleen) should be vaccinated as soon as the diagnosis is made.
  - Pediatric vaccination should be performed according to the recommended pediatric dosage and vaccine types with special consideration made for children less than 2 years of age.
  - When adult vaccination is indicated, the following vaccinations should be administered:
    - ***Streptococcus pneumoniae***
      - Polyvalent pneumococcal vaccine (Pneumovax 23)
    - ***Haemophilus influenzae type B***
      - *Haemophilus influenzae* b vaccine (HibTITER)
    - ***Neisseria meningitidis***
      - Age 16–55: Meningococcal (groups A, C, Y, W-135) polysaccharide diphtheria toxoid conjugate vaccine (Menactra)
      - Age >55: Meningococcal polysaccharide vaccine (Menomune-A/C/Y/W-135)

Vaccine	Dose	Route	Revaccination
Polyvalent pneumococcal	0.5 mL	SC*	Every 6 years
Quadrivalent meningococcal/diphtheria conjugate	0.5 mL	IM upper deltoid	Every 3–5 years†
Quadrivalent meningococcal polysaccharide	0.5 mL	SC*	Every 3–5 years
Hemophilus b conjugate	0.5 mL	IM*	None

*Administered in the deltoid or lateral thigh region.
†Contact the manufacturer for the latest recommendations prior to revaccination.

181. A child had chocolate pastry and got diarrhea within 3 hours of consumption. Which microorganism is responsible for this:

a. S. aureus
b. Pseudomonas
c. Bacillus anthracis
d. Streptococcus

Ans. a. S. aureus

(Ref: Ananthanarayan and Paniker's Textbook of Microbiology 10th edition, page 736)

- S. aureus is also responsible for food poisoning. It is capable of generating toxins that produce food poisoning in the human body.
- Its incubation period lasts one to six hours, with the illness itself lasting from 30 minutes to 3 days. Preventive measures one can take to help prevent the spread of the disease include washing hands thoroughly with soap and water before preparing food.

182. A 27-year-old female with history of PID. She is unable to conceive for last 6 months with unprotected sex. Next step of management is?

a. Hysterosalpingography
b. X-ray
c. MRI
d. USG

Ans. a. Hysterosalpingography

(Ref: DC Dutta's Textbook of Obstetrics 9th edition, page 762)

- Hysterosalpingography (HSG), also known as uterosalpingography, is a radiologic procedure to investigate the shape of the uterine cavity and the shape and patency of the fallopian tubes.
- This means it is a special X-ray using dye to look at the womb (uterus) and Fallopian tubes. It injects a radiopaque material into the cervical canal and usually fluoroscopy with image intensification.

183. Which of the following is most potent anti-oxidant?

a. Vitamin A
b. Vitamin B
c. Vitamin D
d. Vitamin E

Ans. d. Vitamin E *(Ref: Harpers Illustrated Biochemistry 31st edition, page 635)*

- Alpha-tocopherol is the most active form of vitamin E in humans. It is also a powerful biological antioxidant.
- Vitamin E supplements are usually sold as alpha-tocopheryl acetate, a form that protects its ability to function as an antioxidant.

184. Which test is done at subcenter during pregnancy?

a. Hemoglobin
b. B-HCG
c. Amniocentesis
d. All of the above

Ans. a. Hemoglobin

(Ref: Park's Textbook of Preventive and Social Medicine 25th edition, page 635)

- Such a Subcenter having the caseload may be developed as a MCH/type C Subcenter. Antenatal care and Skilled Attendance at Birth by ANMs and LHVs.
- Test for pregnancy confirmation, haemoglobin estimation, urine for albumin and sugar and linkages with PHC for other required tests.

185. Defect seen due to failure of closure of cranial neuropore:

a. Anencephaly
b. Acalvaria
c. Digital amputations
d. Asymmetric ventral wall defects

Ans. a. Anencephaly *(Ref: Robbins Basic Pathology 10th edition, page 625)*

- Failure of closure of the anterior neuropore during embryogenesis will lead to anencephaly, the failure of the brain and skull to develop.
- In less severe situations it may lead to different forms of encephalocele (i.e. cranium bifidum).
- There are three forms of cranium bifidum: meningocele, meningo-encephalocele and meningohydro-encephalocele.
- In which respectively protrude the meninges, the meninges and brain tissue and lastly meninges, brain tissue and cranial ventricles.

186. Evisceration is removal of which coats of eye?

a. Middle
b. Inner layer
c. A + B
d. Sclera shell

Ans. b. Inner layer

(Ref: Comprehensive ophthalmology by AK khurana 7th edition, page 635)

- An evisceration is the removal of the eye's contents, leaving the scleral shell and extraocular muscles intact.
- The procedure is usually performed to reduce pain or improve cosmesis in a blind eye, as in cases of endophthalmitis unresponsive to antibiotics.
- An ocular prosthetic can be fitted over the eviscerated eye in order to improve cosmesis.
- Either general or local anesthetics may be used during eviscerations, with antibiotics and anti-inflammatory agents injected intravenously.

187. Couvelaire uterus is seen in which condition?

a. Abruptio placenta
b. Placenta accreta
c. Placenta praevia
d. Antepartum placenta

Ans. a. Abruptio placenta

(Ref: DC Dutta's Textbook of Obstetrics 9th edition, page 635)

Couvelaire uterus (also known as uteroplacental apoplexy) is a life-threatening condition in which loosening of the placenta (abruptio placentae) causes bleeding that penetrates into the uterine myometrium forcing its way into the peritoneal cavity.

188. The most common cause for PPH is:

a. Trauma
b. Retained tissue
c. Uterine atony
d. Coagulopathy

Ans. c. Uterine atony

(Ref: DC Dutta's Textbook of Obstetrics 9th edition, page 763)

Causes of postpartum hemorrhage

Cause	Incidence
Uterine atony	70%
Trauma	20%
Retained tissue	10%
Coagulopathy	1%

189. A 45-year-old male is brought to casualty after a night party with complain of epigastric pain, penetrating towards back. Which is the best for diagnosis?

a. Serum lipase
b. CPK-MB
c. ALP
d. Gamma-GGT

Ans. a. Serum lipase

(Ref: Harrison's Principles of Internal Medicine 20th edition, vol 2, page 762)

The cardinal symptom of acute pancreatitis is abdominal pain, which is characterized dull, boring and steady.

- Blood tests for lipase may be used to help investigate and diagnose acute pancreatitis and other disorders of the pancreas. Measured serum lipase values may vary depending on the method of analysis.
- Lipase has a slightly longer half-life and its abnormality may support the diagnosis if a delay occurs between the pain episode and the time the patient seeks medical attention.

190. What is the requirement of calories in a woman during lactation in first six months?

a. 600 calories
b. 700 calories
c. 800 calories
d. 1000 calories

Ans. a. 600 calories

(Ref: Park's Textbook of Preventive and Social Medicine 25th edition, page 831)

- **Months 0–6**

  About 170 calories needed each day to produce milk are provided by burning fat leftover from energy stores during pregnancy, and the remaining 500 calories needed must be obtained from the maternal diet. The volume of milk production during the first six months also is the highest, around 780 milliliters per day.
- **Months 7–9**

  By month seven, women need fewer calories while breastfeeding, down to about 400 extra calories each day. This is primarily because the daily volume of milk produced generally decreases during this time to around 600 milliliters per day.

191. What is the hip and pelvic ratio in female and male?

a. 1:1
b. 2:1
c. 0.7:1
d. 0.5:1

Ans. c. 0.7:1

(Ref: Gray's Anatomy 41st edition, page 873)

WHR is used as a measurement of obesity, which in turn is a possible indicator of other more serious health conditions. The WHO states that abdominal obesity is defined as a waist-hip ratio above 0.90 for males and above 0.85 for females, or a body mass index (BMI) above 30.0.

The National Institute of Diabetes, Digestive and Kidney Diseases (NIDDK) states that women with waist-hip ratios of more than 0.8, and men with more than 1.0, are at increased health risk because of their fat distribution.

	DGSP		WHO		NIDDK	
	Women	Men	Women	Men	Women	Men
Under-weight	?	?	?	?	?	?
Normal weight	< 0.80	< 0.90	?	?	?	?
Over-weight	0.80–0.84	0.90–0.99	?	?	?	?
Obesity	> 0.85	> 1.00	> 0.85	> 0.90	> 0.80	> 1.00

192. "Fifth vital sign"commonly elicited by anesthesiologist on surgical patients is:

a. FiO_2 b. Pain
c. Blood pressure d. Core temperature

Ans. b. Pain *(Ref: Morgan and Mikhail's Clinical Anesthesiology, 6th edition, page 635)*

- Pain was officially declared "The Fifth Vital Sign." Henceforth, the evaluation of pain became a requirement of proper patient care as important and basic as the assessment and management of temperature, blood pressure, respiratory rate, and heart rate.
- The numeric pain scale certainly has a place in care and in pain management; however, it is important to assess the patient's communication and self-management style and to recognize that patients, like pain, are on a continuum with varied styles of communication and adaptation.

193. Insecticide of choice for kala-azar:

a. DDT b. Biomagnification
c. Mickey Slim d. Operation Cat Drop

Ans. a. DDT

(Ref: Park's Textbook of Preventive and Social Medicine 25th edition, page 635)

- Indoor residual spraying is a simple and cost effective method of controlling endophilic vectors and DDT remains the insecticide of choice for the control of leishmaniasis.
- However, resistance to insecticide is likely to become more widespread in the population especially in those areas in which insecticide has been used for years.

194. Which of the following is an amplifier host of Japanese encephalitis?

a. Pig b. Dog
c. Human d. Cat

Ans. a. Pig

(Ref: Park's Textbook of Preventive and Social Medicine 25th edition, page 927)

- Pigs act as an amplifying host and have a very important role in the epidemiology of the disease.
- Infection in swine is asymptomatic, except in pregnant sows, when abortion and fetal abnormalities are common sequelae.
- The most important vector is Culex tritaeniorhynchus, which feeds on cattle in preference to humans.
- The natural hosts of the Japanese encephalitis virus are birds, not humans.

195. A person says, I will go home ..... home sweet home, sweet urine? Which of the following condition appropriately describes his condition?

a. Circumstantiality
b. Tangentiality
c. Flow of ideas
d. Derailment

Ans. c. Flow of ideas

(Ref: Diagnostic and Statistical Manual of Mental Disorders 5th edition, page 243)

Flight of ideas describes excessive speech at a rapid rate that involves causal association between ideas. Links between ideas may involve usage of puns or rhymes. It is typical of mania, classically seen in bipolar disorder. Compare derailment.

Circumstantiality (also circumstantial thinking, or circumstantial speech)– An inability to answer a question without giving excessive, unnecessary detail. This differs from tangential thinking, in that the person does eventually return to the original point.

Derailment (also loose association and knight's move thinking)–Thought and/or speech move, either spontaneously or in response to an internal stimulus (distinguishing derailment from "distractible speech," infra), from the topic's track onto another which is obliquely related or unrelated. e.g. "The next day when I'd be going out you know, I took control, like uh, I put bleach on my hair in California."

Tangentiality–Wandering from the topic and never returning to it or providing the information requested. e.g. in answer to the question "Where are you from?", a response "My dog is from England. They have good fish and chips there. Fish breathe through gills."

196. Lumbar puncture is done at which level?

a. L3-L4
b. C3-C4
c. Th12-L1
d. L1-L2

Ans. a. L3-L4 *(Ref: Gray's Anatomy 41st edition, page 635)*

- A lumbar puncture (spinal tap) is the insertion of a needle between the lamina of the vertebrae and into the thecal sac with the purpose of obtaining cerebrospinal fluid.
- This is done below the L2 level (usually between L3-4 or L4-5) in order not to injure the spinal cord.

197. Which of the following is not a premalignant condition?

a. Leukoplakia
b. Erythroplakia
c. Oral submucous fibrosis
d. Aphthous ulcer

Ans. d. Aphthous ulcer

(Ref: Bailey and Love's Short Practice of Surgery, 27th edition, page 736)

The following were identified as Potentially Malignant Disorders by the World Health Organization's working group on Oral Cancer.

- Leukoplakia
- Erythroplakia
- Palatal lesion of reverse cigar smoking
- Oral lichen planus
- Oral submucous fibrosis (SMF)
- Discoid lupus erythematosus.

198. Which organ will be affected most in hypovolemic shock?

a. Liver
b. Lung
c. Kidney
d. Brain

Ans. c. Kidney *(Ref: Bailey and Love's Short Practice of Surgery, 27th edition, page 763)*

Hypovolemic shock as a result of extracellular fluid loss can be of the 4 etiologies

- **Kidney:** Renal losses of salt and fluid can lead to hypovolemic shock. The kidneys usually excrete sodium and water in a manner that matches sodium intake and water intake.
- Diuretic therapy and osmotic diuresis from hyperglycemia can lead to excessive renal sodium and volume loss.
- In addition, there are several tubular and interstitial diseases beyond the scope of this article that cause severe salt-wasting nephropathy.
- Gastrointestinal
- Skin
- Third-spacing

199. Enzymes related to PDH-5 complex:

a. TPP
b. Lipoate
c. Coenzyme A
d. FAD, NAD+

Ans. a. TPP *(Ref: Harpers Illustrated Biochemistry 31st edition, page 736)*

TPP works as a coenzyme in many enzymatic reactions, such as:

- Pyruvate dehydrogenase complex
- Pyruvate decarboxylase in ethanol fermentation
- Alpha-ketoglutarate dehydrogenase complex
- Branched-chain amino acid dehydrogenase complex
- 2-hydroxyphytanoyl-CoA lyase
- Transketolase

200. Which of the following conditions seen with High tracheostomy?

a. Laryngeal carcinoma
b. Neurosurgical patients
c. Spinal cord injury
d. Traumatic brain injury

Ans. a. Laryngeal carcinoma

(Ref: Bailey and Love's Short Practice of Surgery, 27th edition, page 728)

Indications for tracheostomy:

- A. Respiratory obstruction
  - ***Infections:***
    - Acute laryngo-tracheo -bronchitis, acute epiglottitis, diphtheria
    - Ludwig's angina, peritonsillar, retropharyngeal or parapharyngeal abscess, tongue abscess
  - ***Trauma:***
    - External injury of larynx and trachea
    - Trauma due to endoscopies, especially in infants and children
    - Fractures of mandible or maxillofacial injuries
  - ***Neoplasms:***
    - Benign and malignant neoplasms of larynx, pharynx, upper-trachea, tongue and thyroid

- Foreign body larynx
- Edema larynx due to steam, irritant fumes or gases, allergy (angioneurotic or drug sensitivity), radiation
- Bilateral abductor paralysis
- Congenital anomalies:
  - Laryngeal web, cysts, tracheo -esophageal fistula
  - Bilateral choanal atresia.

201. Which of the following route achieved 100% bioavailability?

a. Oral
b. Intravenous
c. Transdermal
d. Subcutaneous

Ans. b. Intravenous

(Ref: Essentials of Medical Pharmacology KDT 8th edition, page 736)

- A drug given by the intravenous route will have an absolute bioavailability of 100% (f = 1), whereas drugs given by other routes usually have an absolute bioavailability of less than one.
- If we compare the two different dosage forms having same active ingredients and compare the two drug bioavailability is called comparative bioavailability.

202. Most common vein used for the central vein infusion:

a. Subclavian
b. Internal jugular vein
c. Axillary vein
d. Femoral vein

Ans. b. Internal jugular vein *(Ref: Gray's Anatomy 41st edition, page 386)*

- A central venous catheter (CVC), also known as a central line, central venous line, or central venous access catheter, is a catheter placed into a large vein. Catheters can be placed in veins in the neck (internal jugular vein), chest (subclavian vein or axillary vein), groin (femoral vein), or through veins in the arms (also known as a PICC line, or peripherally inserted central catheters).
- It is used to administer medication or fluids that are unable to be taken by mouth or would harm a smaller peripheral vein, obtain blood tests (specifically the "central venous oxygen saturation"), and measure central venous pressure.

203. Immunoglobulins are classified on the basis of:

a. Heavy chains (constant region)
b. Light chain (constant domain)
c. Light chain (variable domain)
d. Heave chains (variable region)

Ans. a. Heavy chains (constant region)

(Ref: Robbins Basic Pathology 10th edition, page 672)

Each heavy chain has two regions, the constant region and the variable region. The constant region is identical in all antibodies of the same isotype, but differs in antibodies of different isotypes.

Heavy chains γ, α and δ have a constant region composed of three tandem (in a line) Ig domains, and a hinge region for added flexibility; heavy chains μ and ε have a constant region composed of four immunoglobulin domains.

204. What is the most common symptom of nasopharyngeal carcinoma?

a. Mass in neck/painless/cervical lymphadenopathy
b. Headache
c. Hearning loss
d. Sore throat

Ans. a. Mass in neck/painless/cervical lymphadenopathy

(Ref: Bailey and Love's Short Practice of Surgery, 27th edition, page 526)

- The most common physical finding is a neck mass consisting of painless firm lymph node enlargement (80%).
- Neck involvement is often bilateral; the most common nodes involved are the jugulodigastric, and upper and middle jugular nodes in the anterior cervical chain.
- Possible noticeable symptoms of nasopharyngeal carcinoma include:
  - A lump in your neck caused by a swollen lymph node.
  - Blood in your saliva.
  - Bloody discharge from your nose.
  - Nasal congestion or ringing in your ears.
  - Hearing loss.
  - Frequent ear infections.
  - Sore throat, Headaches.

205. Which of the following organs is not affected in GvHD?

a. Eye
b. Liver
c. Vagina
d. Lung

Ans. a. Eye *(Ref: Bailey and Love's Short Practice of Surgery, 27th edition, page 642)*

- In the classical sense, acute graft-versus-host-disease is characterized by selective damage to the liver, skin (rash), mucosa, and the gastrointestinal tract.
- Newer research indicates that other graft-versus-host-disease target organs include the immune system (the hematopoietic system, e.g. the bone marrow and the thymus) itself, and the lungs in the form of immune-mediated pneumonitis.
- Biomarkers can be used to identify specific causes of GvHD, such as elafin in the skin. Chronic graft-versus-host-disease also attacks the above organs, but over its long-term course can also cause damage to the connective tissue and exocrine glands.
- Mucosal damage to the vagina can result in severe pain and scarring, and appears in both acute and chronic GvHD. This can result in an inability to have sexual intercourse.

206. A person with AB blood group met with RTA. Which blood group he can receive?

a. AB
b. A+ve
c. B+ve
d. All of the above

Ans. d. All of the above

(Ref: Harrison's Principles of Internal Medicine 20th edition, vol 2, page 652)

An individual with type AB blood can receive blood from any group (with AB being preferable), but cannot donate blood to any group other than AB. They are known as universal recipients.

If your blood type is:	You can give to:	You can receive from:
O Positive	O+, A+, B+, AB+	O+, O-
A Positive	A+, AB+	A+, A-, O+, O-
B Positive	B+, AB+	B+, B-, O+, O-
AB Positive	AB+ Only	All blood types

207. Which of the following syndrome is not related to obesity?

a. Bulimia nervosa
b. Prader-Willi syndrome
c. Bardet-Biedl syndrome
d. Cushing's syndrome

Ans. a. Bulimia nervosa

(Ref: Harrison's Principles of Internal Medicine 20th edition, vol 2, page 852)

- Most people with bulimia are at a normal weight. The forcing of vomiting may result in thickened skin on the knuckles and breakdown of the teeth.
- Bulimia is frequently associated with other mental disorders such as depression, anxiety, and problems with drugs or alcohol. All others are related to obesity.

208. What is the precursor of adreno-corticotropic hormone?

a. Cholesterol
b. Bile
c. Acid
d. Triglyceride

Ans. a. Cholesterol *(Ref: Harpers Illustrated Biochemistry 31st edition, page 626)*

- The rapid actions of ACTH include stimulation of cholesterol delivery to the mitochondria where the P450 scc enzyme is located. P450 scc catalyzes the first step of steroidogenesis that is cleavage of the side-chain of cholesterol.
- ACTH also stimulates lipoprotein uptake into cortical cells. This increases the bioavailability of cholesterol in the cells of the adrenal cortex.

209. What is most common complication after stripping of varicose veins?

a. Ecchymosis
b. Petechia
c. Pigmented purpuric dermatosis
d. Purpura

Ans. a. Ecchymosis

(Ref: Bailey and Love's Short Practice of Surgery, 27th edition, page 1538)

- Stripping consists of removal of all or part the saphenous vein (great/long or lesser/short) main trunk. The complications include deep vein thrombosis (5.3%), pulmonary embolism (0.06%), and wound complications including infection (2.2%).
- There is evidence for the great saphenous vein regrowing after stripping. For traditional surgery, reported recurrence rates, which have been tracked for 10 years, range from 5–60%. In addition, since stripping removes the saphenous main trunks, they are no longer available for use as venous bypass grafts in the future (coronary or leg artery vital disease).
- Leg symptoms were defined as pain, itching, muscle cramps, throbbing, and swelling. Ulcers, pigmentations and ecchymosis were recorded as signs of varicose vein. Ecchymosis was defined as a hemorrhagic lesions, larger than >3 mm on the skin of lower extremities, forming a flat, rounded or irregular, blue or purplish patch.

210. Pregnancy for how many times will be considered as grand parity?

a. 5 times
b. 7 times
c. 9 times
d. 10 times

Ans. a. 5 times *(Ref: DC Dutta's Textbook of Obstetrics 9th edition, page 653)*

A reasonable definition of "grand multiparity" is a woman who has had ≥5 births (live or stillborn) at ≥20 weeks of gestation, with "great grand multiparity" defined as ≥10 births (live or stillborn) ≥20 weeks of gestation. However, other definitions are also used.

211. Which of the following is the best community health indicator?

a. IMR
b. MMR
c. Life expectancy
d. Proportional mortality rate

Ans. a. IMR

(Ref: Park's Textbook of Preventive and Social Medicine 25th edition, page 955)

- The infant mortality rate is the number of infant deaths for every 1,000 live births.
- In addition to giving us key information about maternal and infant health, the infant mortality rate is an important marker of the overall health of a society.
- MR remains an important indicator of health for whole populations, reflecting the intuition that structural factors affecting the health of entire populations have an impact on the mortality rate of infants.

212. Which of the following is to be done in bio-medical waste management?

a. Incinerated
b. Burn pit
c. Cremation
d. Gasification

Ans. a. Incinerated

(Ref: Park's Textbook of Preventive and Social Medicine 25th edition, page 763)

- The goals of biomedical waste treatment are to reduce or eliminate the waste's hazards, and usually to make the waste unrecognizable.
- Treatment should render the waste safe for subsequent handling and disposal. There are several treatment methods that can accomplish these goals.
- Biomedical waste is often incinerated. An efficient incinerator will destroy pathogens and sharps. Source materials are not recognizable in the resulting ash.
- Alternative thermal treatment can also include technologies such as gasification and pyrolysis including energy recovery with similar waste volume reductions and pathogen destruction.

213. If radius of vein becomes double, blood flow will be increased by how many times?

a. 16 times
b. 20 times
c. 24 times
d. 28 times

Ans. a. 16 times *(Ref: Guyton and Hall 13th edition, page 548)*

- A lumen diameter on resistance is dramatic: A slight increase or decrease in diameter causes a huge decrease or increase in resistance. This is because resistance is inversely proportional to the radius of the blood vessel (one-half of the vessel's diameter) raised to the fourth power ($R = 1/r^4$).

- This means, e.g. that if an artery or arteriole constricts to one-half of its original radius, the resistance to flow will increase 16 times. And if an artery or arteriole dilates to twice its initial radius, then resistance in the vessel will decrease to 1/16 of its original value and flow will increase 16 times.

214. Which prostaglandin is used in labor induction?

a. Prostaglandin E2 (PGE2)
b. Prostaglandin E1 analog (PGE1)
c. Prostaglandin $F_{2\alpha}$ ($PGF_{2\alpha}$)
d. All of the above

Ans. d. All of the above

(Ref: Essentials of Medical Pharmacology KDT 8th edition, page 752)

Pharmacological methods include dinoprostone (prostaglandin E2), misoprostol (a prostaglandin E1 analog).

- Prostaglandin E2 (PGE2), also known as dinoprostone, is a naturally occurring prostaglandin which is used as a medication. As a medication it is used in labor induction
- Misoprostol is a synthetic prostaglandin E1 analog that is used off-label for a variety of indications in the practice of obstetrics and gynecology, including medication abortion, medical management of miscarriage, induction of labor, cervical ripening before surgical procedures, and the treatment of postpartum hemorrhage
- Prostaglandin $F_{2\alpha}$ ($PGF_{2\alpha}$ in prostanoid nomenclature), pharmaceutically termed carboprost, is a naturally occurring prostaglandin used in medicine to induce labor and as an abortifacient.

215. De novo synthesis of fatty acid requires which coenzyme (HCL)?

a. FAD
b. NAD
c. NADPH
d. TPP

Ans. c. NADPH *(Ref: Harpers Illustrated Biochemistry 31st edition, page 327)*

De novo fatty acid synthesis:

- Fatty acid are synthesized by an extra mitochondrial system.
- Acetyl-CoA is the immediate substrate, and free palmitate is the end product.
- It's cofactor and coenzymes include NADPH, ATP, Mn^{+2}, Biotin, HCO^{3}_{-}
- NADPH is donor of reducing equivalents.

216. Which of the following is feature of hairy cell leukemia?

a. Cladribine is C/I
b. Malignant B lymphocytes
c. High platelet count
d. Low lymphocyte counts

Ans. b. Malignant B lymphocytes

(Ref: Harrison's Principles of Internal Medicine 20th edition, vol 2, page 873)

The "hairy cells" (malignant B lymphocytes) accumulate in the bone marrow, interfering with the production of normal white blood cells, red blood cells, and platelets. Consequently, patients may develop infections related to low white blood cell count, anemia and fatigue due to a lack of red blood cells, or easy bleeding due to a low platelet count.

Pancytopenia in HCL is caused primarily by marrow failure and splenomegaly. Bone marrow failure is caused by the accumulation of hairy cells and reticulin fibrosis in the bone marrow, as well as by the detrimental effects of dysregulated cytokine production.

A complete blood count (CBC) normally shows low counts for white blood cells, red blood cells, and platelets in HCL patients. However, if large numbers of hairy cells are in the blood stream, then normal or even high lymphocyte counts may be found.

Cladribine (2CDA) and pentostatin (DCF) are the two most common first-line therapies. They both belong to a class of medications called purine analogs, which have mild side effects compared to traditional chemotherapy regimens.

217. Prevention of emerging risk factors of coronary artery disease is what level of prevention?

a. Primary
b. Secondary
c. Tertiary
d. Primordial

Ans. d. Primordial

(Ref: Park's Textbook of Preventive and Social Medicine 25th edition, page 341)

Level of prevention	Modes of intervention
Primordial	Before emergence of risk factor
Primary	Health promotion and specific protection
Sec	Early diagnosis and treatment
Tertiary	Disability limitation and rehabilitation

218. Praziquantel is used to treat all disease *except*:

a. Hydatid disease
b. Fluke infections
c. Tapeworm infection
d. Ocular cysticercosis

Ans. d. Ocular cysticercosis

(Ref: Comprehensive Ophthalmology by AK Khurana 7th edition, page 446)

- Praziquantel (PZQ), sold under the brandname Biltricide among others, is a medication used to treat a number of types of parasitic worm infections.
- Specifically it is used for schistosomiasis, clonorchiasis, opisthorchiasis, tapeworm infections, cysticercosis, hydatid disease, and other fluke infections.
- Parasite destruction within the eye may cause irreversible lesions, ocular cysticercosis must not be treated with this compound.

219. The objective of RNTCP program is as follows:

a. Cure rate 85%
b. Case detection rate over 70%
c. Both
d. Cure rate 95%

Ans. c. Both

(Ref: Park's Textbook of Preventive and Social Medicine 25th edition, page 451)

- The program has developed a strategic vision for TB control for the country up to 2015, under which it aims to achieve and maintain a cure rate of at least 85% in new sputum-positive (NSP) pulmonary TB patients and achieve detection rates of such cases of at least 70%.
- The RNTCP has sustained the objectives (NSP case detection rates of over 70% and treatment success rates of over 85% nationally) since 2007, in line with global targets for TB control.

220. Dialation of pupils seen in:

a. Horner's syndrome
b. Intracranial hemorrhage
c. Hereditary disorders
d. Epilepsy

Ans. d. Epilepsy

(Ref: Comprehensive Ophthalmology by AK Khurana 7th edition, page 346)

Mydriasis is the dilation of the pupil, usually having a non-physiological cause, or sometimes a physiological pupillary response. Non-physiological causes of mydriasis include disease, trauma, or the use of drugs.

Multiple central nervous system disorders, e.g. epilepsy, stroke, and impending brain herniation are known to lead to temporal mydriasis as well. A brain catastrophe, or a rapidly increasing brain mass, can cause compression of the oculomotor nerve.

Miosis or myosis is excessive constriction of the pupil:

- Senile miosis (a reduction in the size of a person's pupil in old age
- Horner's syndrome
- Hemorrhage into pons (intracranial hemorrhage)
- Hereditary disorders
- Cluster headache with ptosis
- Iridocyclitis
- Fatal familial insomnia.

221. Poliovirus can be detected in specimens from:

a. Feces stool sample
b. Throat
c. Cerebrospinal fluid
d. All of the above

Ans. d. All of the above

(Ref: Ananthanarayan and Paniker's Textbook of Microbiology 10th edition, page 272)

Poliovirus can be detected in specimens from the throat, and feces (stool), and occasionally cerebrospinal fluid (CSF), by isolating the virus in cell culture or by detecting the virus by polymerase chain reaction (PCR).

CDC laboratories conduct testing for poliovirus including:

- Culture
- Intratypic differentiation
- Genome sequencing
- Serology.

222. Which of the following is wound care agent among the following?

a. Hypochlorous acid
b. Dichlorine monoxide
c. Hypofluorous acid
d. Perchloric acid

Ans. a. Hypochlorous acid

(Ref: Bailey & Love's Short Practice of Surgery, 27th edition, page 563)

- Hypochlorous acid has been investigated as a possible wound care agent, and as of early 2016 the US. Food and Drug Administration has approved products whose main active ingredient is hypochlorous acid for use in treating wounds and various infections in humans and pets. It is also FDA-approved as a preservative for saline solutions.

- In organic synthesis, hypochlorous acid (HClO) converts alkenes to chlorohydrins.
- In biology, HClO is generated in activated neutrophils by myeloperoxidase-mediated peroxidation of chloride ions, and contributes to the destruction of bacteria.

223. All of the following are true about ECG myocardial infarction *except*:

a. ST elevation
b. Tall T wave
c. Hypokalemia
d. Q waves

Ans. c. Hypokalemia

(Ref: Harrison's Principles of Internal Medicine 20th edition, vol 1, page 738)

- The earliest presentation of acute myocardial infarction is the hyperacute T wave, which is treated the same as ST segment elevation. In practice this is rarely seen, because it only exists for 2–30 minutes after the onset of infarction. Hyperacute T waves need to be distinguished from the peaked T waves associated with hyperkalemia.
- In the first few hours the ST segments usually begin to rise. Pathological Q waves may appear within hours or may take greater than 24 hr. The T wave will generally become inverted in the first 24 hours, as the ST elevation begins to resolve.
- Long-term changes of ECG include persistent Q waves (in 90% of cases) and persistent inverted T waves. Persistent ST elevation is rare except in the presence of a ventricular aneurysm.

224. Cheyne–Stokes is abnormal pattern states the abnormality of:

a. Nerves
b. Breathing
c. Pumping
d. Excretion

Ans. b. Breathing *(Ref: Robbins Basic Pathology 10th edition, page 273)*

- Cheyne–Stokes respiration is an abnormal pattern of breathing characterized by progressively deeper, and sometimes faster, breathing followed by a gradual decrease that results in a temporary stop in breathing called an apnea.
- The pattern repeats, with each cycle usually taking 30 seconds to 2 minutes.
- It is an oscillation of ventilation between apnea and hyperpnea with a crescendo-diminuendo pattern, and is associated with changing serum partial pressures of oxygen and carbon dioxide.

225. Most common causes of postpartum hemorrhage:

a. Uterine atony
b. Trauma
c. Retained tissue
d. Coagulopathy

Ans. a. Uterine atony *(Ref: DC Dutta's Textbook of Obstetrics 9th edition, page 295)*

Causes of postpartum hemorrhage	
Cause	**Incidence**
Uterine atony	70%
Trauma	20%
Retained tissue	10%
Coagulopathy	1%

Causes of postpartum hemorrhage are uterine atony, trauma, retained placenta or placental abnormalities, and coagulopathy, commonly referred to as the "four Ts".

226. All of the following is true about Thermoactinomycetaceae *except*:

a. Gram-negative
b. Endospore-forming
c. Bacteria
d. Prokaryotic

Ans. a. Gram-negative

(Ref: Ananthanarayan and Paniker's Textbook of Microbiology 10th edition, page 652)

The Thermoactinomycetaceae are a family of Gram-positive endospore-forming bacteria. They are Prokaryotic.

227. Night blindness is caused by:

a. VIT A
b. VIT B
c. VIT C
d. VIT D

Ans. a. VIT A

(Ref: Robbins Basic Pathology 10th edition, page 407)

- Vitamin A deficiency (VAD) or hypovitaminosis A is a lack of vitamin A in blood and tissues. It is common in poorer countries, but rarely is seen in more developed countries. Nyctalopia (night blindness) is one of the first signs of VAD.
- Xerophthalmia, keratomalacia, and complete blindness can also occur since vitamin A has a major role in phototransduction.
- The three forms of vitamin A include retinols, beta-carotenes, and carotenoids.

228. Prader–Willi syndrome is a caused by loss of function of genes in a particular region of chromosome:

a. Chromosome 10
b. Chromosome 15
c. Chromosome 18
d. Chromosome 21

Ans. b. Chromosome 15 *(Ref: Robbins Basic Pathology 10th edition, page 339)*

Prader-Willi syndrome is caused by the loss of function of genes in a particular region of chromosome 15 located in the region 15q11–13. People normally inherit one copy of this chromosome from each parent. Some genes are turned on (active) only on the copy that is inherited from a person's father (the paternal copy).

229. Commotio retinae is also knows as:

a. Berlin's edema
b. Traumatic maculopathy
c. Pedal edema
d. Peripheral edema

Ans. a. Berlin's edema

(Ref: Comprehensive Ophthalmology by AK Khurana 7th edition, page 262)

- Berlin's edema (commotio retinae) a common condition caused by blunt injury to the eye.
- It is characterized by decreased vision in the injured eye a few hours after the injury.
- Under examination the retina appears opaque and white in color in the periphery but the blood vessels are normally seen along with "cherry red spot" in the foveal region.

- The choroidal fluorescence in fluorescent angiography is absent. Visual acuity ranges from 20/20 to 20/400.

230. Undercooked fish infection is caused by:

a. Diphyllobothriasis
b. Rouphozoa
c. Platyhelminthes
d. Anisakiasis

Ans. a. Diphyllobothriasis

(Ref: Ananthanarayan and Paniker's Textbook of Microbiology 10th edition, page 447)

- A fish tapeworm infection can occur when a person eats raw or undercooked fish that's contaminated with the parasite Diphyllobothrium latum.
- The parasite is more commonly known as the fish tapeworm.
- This type of tapeworm grows in hosts such as small organisms in the water and large mammals that eat raw fish.
- It's passed through the feces of animals. A person becomes infected after ingesting improperly prepared freshwater fish that contain tapeworm cysts.

231. Antibiotic prior to surgery is given at what time?

a. 10 minutes
b. 30 minutes
c. 2 hours
d. 4 hours

Ans. b. 30 minutes

(Ref: Morgan and Mikhail's Clinical Anesthesiology, 6th edition, page 177)

- Timing of antibiotic administration is critical to efficacy.
- The first dose should always be given before the procedure, preferably within 30 minutes before incision.
- Readministration at one to two half-lives of the antibiotic is recommended for the duration of the procedure.

232. New drug testing to compare with existing drug:

a. Statistical inference
b. Random control trial
c. Drug development
d. Hypothesis testing

Ans. a. Statistical inference

(Ref: Morgan and Mikhail's Clinical Anesthesiology, 6th edition, page 253)

- Randomized control trial (RCT) is a type of scientific (often medical) experiment that aims to reduce certain sources of bias when testing the effectiveness of new treatments; this is accomplished by randomly allocating subjects to two or more groups, treating them differently, and then comparing them with respect to a measured response.
- One group—the experimental group—has the intervention being assessed, while the other—usually called the control group—has an alternative condition, such as a placebo or no intervention.
- The groups are followed under conditions of the trial design to see how effective the experimental intervention was.
- Treatment efficacy is assessed in comparison to the control. There may be more than one treatment group or more than one control group.

233. All of the following are true about Salmonella *except*:

a. XLD agar
b. Pike's medium
c. Produce hydrogen sulphide
d. Sugar fermentation

Ans. a. XLD agar

(Ref: Ananthanarayan and Paniker's Textbook of Microbiology 10th edition, page 345)

- Xylose lysine deoxycholate agar (XLD agar) is a selective growth medium used in the isolation of Salmonella and Shigella species from clinical samples and from food.
- Most gut bacteria, including Salmonella, can ferment the sugar xylose to produce acid.
- Salmonella metabolize thiosulfate to produce hydrogen sulfide, which leads to the formation of colonies with black centers and allows them to be differentiated from the similarly colored Shigella colonies.
- Pike's Media: Preservation of *S. pyogenes*, pneumococci, and *Haemophilus influenzae* in nose and throat swabs.

234. Which of the following is example of blood stain test?

a. Hemin crystal
b. Gram stain
c. Both
d. None

Ans. a. Hemin crystal *(Ref: Guyton and Hall 13th edition, page 524)*

- Ludwig Karl Teichmann was a Polish anatomist and physician who made an enduring contribution to forensic science with his discovery of the Teichmann test for hemoglobin. Also called the Teichmann crystal, this is a test that is used on dried stains to determine whether or not blood is present.
- Dr. Teichmann made his forensic discovery in 1853. His microcrystalline test remains in use today as a means of identifying whether or not dried stains at a crime scene, on clothing or other fabric, or elsewhere at the site of a forensic investigation contain (human) blood.

235. A female patient feels that her intestine is rotten. Which psychiatric illness she is suffering from?

a. Munchausen syndrome
b. Nocebo
c. Somatoform disorder
d. Medically unexplained physical symptoms

Ans. c. Somatoform disorder

(Ref: Diagnostic and Statistical Manual of Mental Disorders 5th edition, page 248)

- Somatoform disorder, is any mental disorder that manifests as physical symptoms that suggest illness or injury, but cannot be explained fully by a general medical condition or by the direct effect of a substance, and are not attributable to another mental disorder (e.g. panic disorder) Somatic symptom disorders, as a group, are included in a number of diagnostic schemes of mental illness.

236. She think she had a heart attack pain prolonged for 20 minutes:

a. Panic attack
b. Nervous breakdown
c. Social anxiety disorder
d. Post-traumatic stress disorder

Ans. a. Panic attack

(Ref: Diagnostic and Statistical Manual of Mental Disorders 5th edition, page 234)

- Panic attacks are sudden periods of intense fear that may include palpitations, sweating, shaking, shortness of breath, numbness, or a feeling that something bad is going to happen.
- The maximum degree of symptoms occurs within minutes.
- Typically they last for about 30 minutes but the duration can vary from seconds to hours. There may be a fear of losing control or chest pain. Panic attacks themselves are not typically dangerous physical.

237. SNHL (sensorineural hearing loss) cochlear implant in infant is:

a. BAHA
b. SAHA
c. DAHA
d. FAHA

Ans. a. BAHA *(Ref: Dhingra's Diseases of ENT 7th edition, page 342)*

- The Bone Anchored Hearing Aid (BAHA) is a surgically implanted device designed to help people with hearing loss.
- The majority of the conventional hearing aids transmit sound through the medium of air conduction. BAHA stimulates the cochlea by transmitting the sound waves through the bones in our skull, or bone conduction, thereby bypassing the outer and middle ear.
- Once the cochlea receives the sound signals, the information is converted in to neural signals and transferred to the brain, where it is perceived as sound. Thereby bypassing the outer and middle ear.

238. Level of scapula is at:

a. T3
b. T4
c. T6
d. T7

Ans. d. T7 *(Ref: Gray's Anatomy 41st edition, page 253)*

- The vertebral levels summarized below are useful. The spinous processes of the C6 and 7 and T1 vertebra are usually visible in vivo when the neck is flexed. The apex of the lung and the cupola of the pleura extend to the C7 vertebral level.
- The spine of the scapula is commonly in line with the T3 vertebra, and the manubrium of the sternum is generally opposite T3 and 4 vertebra.
- The trachea divides at the level of vertebra T5 to 7 when a subject is in the erect position. The inferior angle of the scapula is frequently at the level of the spinous process of the T7 vertebra.
- The xiphisternal junction is approximately opposite the T10 vertebra. The spinal cord usually ends at the L1 or 2 vertebral level.
- The supracristal plane (through the highest points of the iliac crests), which is typically at the L4 vertebral level, is used as a landmark for lumbar puncture, and the aorta divides at this level.
- The anterior and posterior superior iliac spines (the latter being frequently marked by a dimple) are at the level of the second sacral segment.

239. Farmer's infection of food is:

a. Madura foot
b. Malignant neoplasm
c. Tropical ulcer
d. Leprosy

Ans. a. Madura foot

(Ref: Ananthanarayan and Paniker's Textbook of Microbiology 10th edition, page 535)

- The disease is usually seen in field workers like farmers, and generally affects men between 20 years and 40 years.
- Eumycetoma is a chronic granulomatous fungal disease of humans, affecting mainly the limbs, and sometimes the abdominal and chest walls or the head.
- Mycetoma pedis (mycetoma of the foot), the most common form of mycetoma, is known widely as the Madura foot.

240. Normal fasting blood sugar level:

a. 100 mg/dL
b. 110 mg/dL
c. 120 mg/dL
d. 130 mg/dL

Ans. a. 100 mg/dL *(Ref: Guyton and Hall 13th edition, page 142)*

- Fasting blood sugar test. A blood sample will be taken after an overnight fast. A fasting blood sugar level less than 100 mg/dL (5.6 mmol/L) is normal.
- A fasting blood sugar level from 100 to 125 mg/dL (5.6 to 6.9 mmol/L) is considered prediabetes.
- If it's 126 mg/dL (7 mmol/L) or higher on two separate tests, you have diabetes.

241. Which is the upper limit of initiation of first dose of rotavirus?

a. 5 weeks
b. 10 weeks
c. 15 weeks
d. 20 weeks

Ans. c. 15 weeks

(Ref: OP Ghai Pediatrics 10th edition, page 251)

- Advisory committee on immunization practices (ACIP) recommends vaccination of preterm infants according to the same schedule and precautions as full-term infants. In preterm infants (as in full-term infants), the maximum chronological age for the first dose is 14 weeks 6 days.
- Vaccination should not be initiated for infants aged 15 weeks 0 days or older because of insufficient data on safety of dose 1 of rotavirus vaccine in older infants.

242. A term baby is apneic and has a heart rate 90/min. Bag and mask ventilation was given for 30 seconds. Subsequently the heart rate is still less than 100 bpm. What is the next step?

a. Give chest compression
b. Give supplemental oxygen
c. Check chest movement
d. Reduce oxygen supply

Ans. c. Check chest movement *(Ref: OP Ghai Pediatrics 10th edition, page 372)*

Since 30 seconds of PPV has already been administered and heart rate is still less than 100 bpm, check chest movement to take ventilation corrective steps.

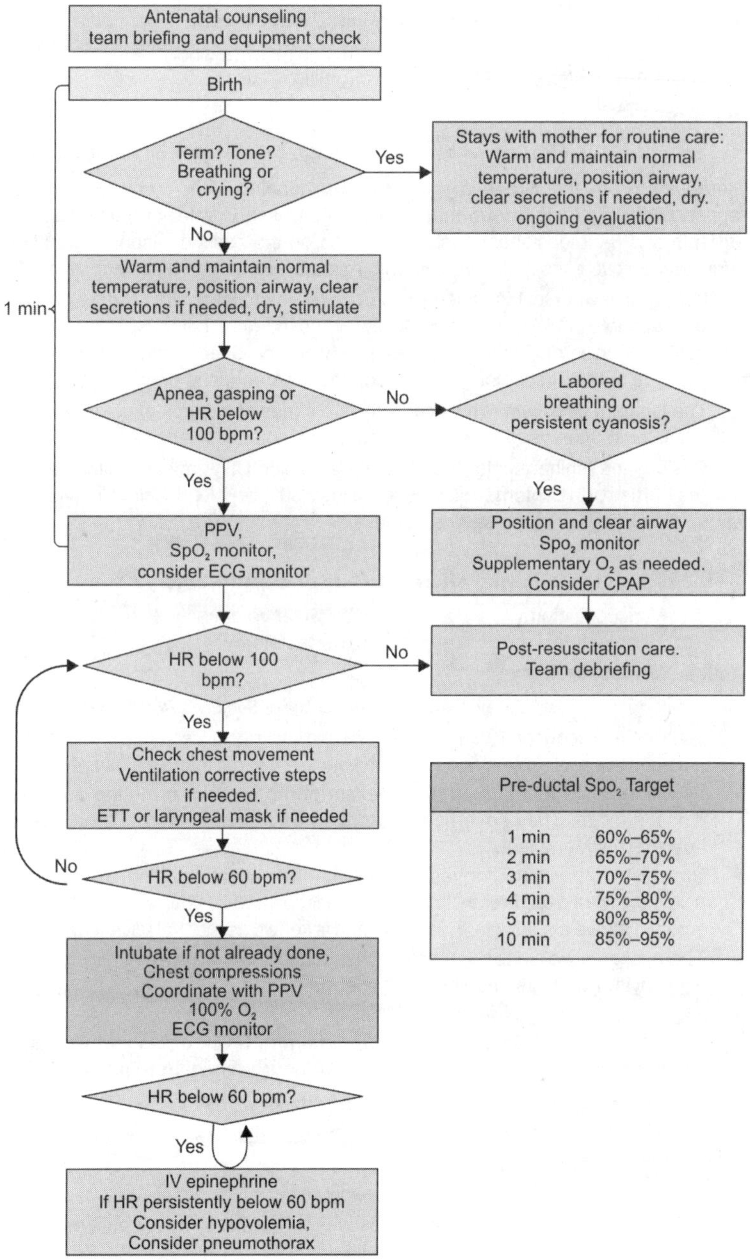
Antenatal counseling
team briefing and equipment check
Birth
Term? Tone? Breathing or crying?
Yes
Stays with mother for routine care: Warm and maintain normal temperature, position airway, clear secretions if needed, dry. ongoing evaluation
No
Warm and maintain normal temperature, position airway, clear secretions if needed, dry, stimulate
1 min
Apnea, gasping or HR below 100 bpm?
No
Labored breathing or persistent cyanosis?
Yes
Yes
PPV, SpO2 monitor, consider ECG monitor
Position and clear airway
Spo2 monitor
Supplementary O2 as needed.
Consider CPAP
HR below 100 bpm?
No
Post-resuscitation care.
Team debriefing
Yes
Check chest movement
Ventilation corrective steps if needed.
ETT or laryngeal mask if needed
Pre-ductal Spo2 Target
1 min 60%–65%
2 min 65%–70%
3 min 70%–75%
4 min 75%–80%
5 min 80%–85%
10 min 85%–95%
No
HR below 60 bpm?
Yes
Intubate if not already done,
Chest compressions
Coordinate with PPV
100% O2
ECG monitor
HR below 60 bpm?
Yes
IV epinephrine
If HR persistently below 60 bpm
Consider hypovolemia,
Consider pneumothorax

243. All of the following are color blindness test *except*:

a. Ishihara
b. Holmgren's wool
c. Farnsworth Lantern Test
d. Stereopsis

Ans. d. Stereopsis

(Ref: Comprehensive Ophthalmology by AK Khurana 7th edition, page 438)

Stereopsis (from the Greek στερεο- stereo- meaning "solid", and ὄψις opsis, "appearance, sight") is a term that is most often used to refer to the perception of depth and 3-dimensional structure obtained on the basis of visual information deriving from two eyes by individuals with normally developed binocular vision.

Holmgren's wool test is based on the principles of Helmholtz's theory of color vision. Helmholtz (1866) had tentatively proposed that color blindness could manifest itself in three forms--red, green, or violet blindness—depending on the missing type of color receptor (one for red, one for green, and one for violet).

The Ishihara color test, which consists of a series of pictures of colored spots, is the test most often used to diagnose red–green color deficiencies.

Besides the Ishihara color test, the US Navy and US Army also allow testing with the Farnsworth Lantern Test. This test allows 30% of color deficient individuals, whose deficiency is not too severe, to pass.

244. Which of the following referred to bag of worms surgery?

a. Varicocelectomy
b. Splenectomy
c. Hepatectomy
d. Rectotomy

Ans. a. Varicocelectomy

(Ref: Bailey & Love's Short Practice of Surgery, 27th edition, page 438)

- Varicocele, pronounced "vari-co-seel," is when veins in your scrotum swell and get enlarged. It's a lot like a varicose vein in your leg. It might feel like a bag of worms.
- Varicoceles are found through self-exam of the scrotum or during a routine doctor's exam. They have been described as a "bag of worms" because of how they look and feel.
- Urologists often check for varicoceles with the patient standing. You may be asked to take a deep breath, hold it, and bear down while your urologist feels the scrotum above the testicle. This technique is known as the "Valsalva maneuver."
- There is tentative evidence that varicocelectomy may improve fertility in those with obvious findings and abnormal sperm.

245. A patient came into emergency complaining fever, chills and swelling in right-upper-quadrant (RUQ), the most porbable diagnosis:

a. Biliary disease
b. Cholecystitis
c. Hepatocellular carcinoma
d. Liver abscess

Ans. d. Liver abscess

(Ref: Harrison's Principles of Internal Medicine 20th edition, vol 2, page 1392)

- The clinical presentation of liver abscess is insidious; many patients have symptoms for weeks before presentation.
- Fever and RUQ pain are the most common complaints. Pain is reported in as many as 80% of patients and may be associated with pleuritic chest pain or right shoulder pain.

- Symptoms are often misdiagnosed as acute cholecystitis. Fever occurs in 87–100% of patients and is usually associated with chills and malaise.

246. Subperiosteal hemorrhage in the long bones is usually seen in:

a. Scurvy
b. Rickets
c. Hemophillia
d. Osteogenesis imperfecta

Ans. a. Scurvy *(Ref: Rockwood and Green's Fractures in Adults 8th edition, page 97)*

Scurvy is a result of insufficient dietary intake of vitamin C, which is required for collagen synthesis. Clinical manifestations include mucous membrane bleeding, orbital hemorrhage, and subperiosteal hemorrhage (especially in infants).

247. LOOK to see if the skin pinch goes back very slowly, The next step to be done is:

a. ORS after every episode of diarrhea
b. ORS after every second episode of diarrhea
c. ORS after every third episode of diarrhoea
d. No ORS at all

Ans. a. ORS after every episode of diarrhea

(Ref: Ananthanarayan and Paniker's Textbook of Microbiology 10th edition, page 427)

- Babies may be given ORS with a dropper or a syringe. Infants under two may be given a teaspoon of ORS fluid every one to two minutes. Older children and adults should take frequent sips from a cup, with a recommended intake of 200–400 mL of solution after every loose movement.
- WHO recommends giving children under two a quarter- to a half-cup of fluid following each loose bowel movement and older children a half- to a full cup. If the person vomits, the caretaker should wait 5–10 minutes and then resume giving ORS.

248. All are seen in congenital rubella syndrome *except*:

a. Sensorineural deafness
b. Glaucoma
c. Pulmonary artery stenosis
d. Headlight in fog appearance

Ans. d. Headlight in fog appearance

(Ref: Ananthanarayan and Paniker's Textbook of Microbiology 10th edition, page 342)

The classic triad for congenital rubella syndrome is:

- Sensorineural deafness (58% of patients)
- Eye abnormalities—especially retinopathy, cataract, glaucoma, and microphthalmia (43% of patients)
- Congenital heart disease—especially pulmonary artery stenosis and patent ductus arteriosus (50% of patients).

249. All of the following are fat-soluble vitamins *except*:

a. VIT A
b. VIT B12
c. VIT D
d. VIT E

Ans. b. VIT B12 *(Ref: Harpers Illustrated Biochemistry 31st edition, page 354)*

- Vitamins are classified as either water-soluble or fat-soluble.
- In humans there are 13 vitamins: 4 fat-soluble (A, D, E, and K) and 9 water-soluble (8 B vitamins and vitamin C).

250. Most radio-exposure is seen with which of the following investigation?

a. IVP b. X-ray
c. USG d. MRI

Ans. a. IVP *(Ref: The Basics and Fundamentals of imaging 4th edition, page 232)*

IVP is most radio exposure among the following:

- If kidney impairment is found before administration of the contrast, metformin should be stopped 48 hours before and after the procedure.
- Contrast allergy: If the patient has any previous history of adverse or moderate reactions to contrast medium.
- Patient with significantly decreased kidney function; because contrast media can be nephrotoxic and worsen kidney function.

251. Which of the following disease common after disaster malaria?

a. Gastroenteritis b. Appendicitis
c. Volvulus d. Inflammatory bowel disease

Ans. a. Gastroenteritis

(Ref: Park's Textbook of Preventive and Social Medicine 25th edition, page 638)

- Regarding diarrheal diseases (the most reported diseases in post-disaster settings), it is important to emphasize that rehydration therapy remains the same for any etiology of acute gastroenteritis and should start as soon as possible before the results of other investigations are obtained.
- We recommend re-establishing and improving the delivery of primary healthcare through restoration of affected health services. Besides a sufficient level of sanitation, medical supplies should be provided and training of healthcare workers and medical personnel on appropriate case management should be conducted.

252. Anemia of a community is best studied by which study?

a. Case–control study b. Cross-sectional
c. Longitudinal study d. Cohort studies

Ans. b. Cross-sectional

(Ref: Park's Textbook of Preventive and Social Medicine 25th edition, page 462)

- We conducted a combined study of rural adults 18–64 years of age with a repeated cross-sectional component (4456 in 2006 and 2184 in 2008) and a cohort component (1424) in rural Deqing, China.
- Anemia was diagnosed based on blood hemoglobin levels using the hemiglobincyanide (HiCN) method according to both the WHO and Chinese criteria.
- The prevalence and incidence of anemia and their 95% confidential intervals (95% CI) were calculated.

253. A definitive diagnosis of gout is based upon the identification of uric acid in:

a. Blood
b. Cerebrospinal fluid
c. Synovial fluid
d. Urine

Ans. c. Synovial fluid

(Ref: Harpers Illustrated Biochemistry 31st edition, page 495)

- Indefinitive diagnosis of gout is based upon the identification of monosodium urate crystals in synovial fluid or a tophus.
- All synovial fluid samples obtained from undiagnosed inflamed joints by arthrocentesis should be examined for these crystals.
- Under polarized light microscopy, they have a needle-like morphology and strong negative birefringence.

254. Which of the following is true about ranula?

a. Retension cyst of sublingual gland
b. Retension cyst of submandibular gland
c. Extravasation cyst of sublingual gland
d. Extravasation cyst of submandibular gland

Ans. c. Extravasation cyst of sublingual gland

(Ref: Dhingra's Diseases of ENT 7th edition, Page 293)

- A ranula is a mucus extravasation cyst involving a sublingual gland and is a type of mucocele found on the floor of the mouth.
- Ranula present as a swelling of connective tissue consisting of collected mucin from a ruptured salivary gland caused by local trauma.

255. McArdle disease is caused by deficiency of:

a. Muscle phosphorylase
b. Phosphorylase
c. Kinase mcat
d. None

Ans. a. Muscle phosphorylase

(Ref: Robbins Basic Pathology 10th edition, page 488)

- McArdle disease is a deficiency of muscle phosphorylase. This is an important substance needed to break down glycogen in your muscle cells.
- The condition causes fatigue and muscle pain during exercise. The disease can lead to dark urine.

256. Nonmalignant lesion of mouth is:

a. Aphthous ulcer
b. Malignant ulcer
c. Oral candidiasis
d. Herpes labialis

Ans. a. Aphthous ulcer

(Ref: Robbins Basic Pathology 10th edition, page 203)

- Aphthous stomatitis is a common condition characterized by the repeated formation of benign and non-contagious mouth ulcers (aphthae) in otherwise healthy individuals.
- The informal term canker sores is also used, mainly in North America, although this may also refer to any mouth ulcers.

257. The secretory phase is starts on which day of menstruation cycle?

a. 1st day
b. 4th day
c. 14th day
d. 24th day

Ans. c. 14th day *(Ref: Guyton and Hall 13th edition, page 543)*

- The first phase of the menstrual cycle is the follicular or proliferative phase. It occurs from day zero to day 14 of the menstrual cycle, based on the average duration of 28 days.
- Ovulation always occurs 14 days before menses; therefore, with an average 28 day cycle, ovulation occurs on day 14.
- The next phase of the menstrual cycle is the luteal or secretory phase. This phase always occurs from day 14 to day 28 of the cycle.
- Progesterone stimulated by LH is the dominant hormone during this phase to prepare the corpus luteum and the endometrium for possible fertilized ovum implantation.

258. Extrinsic pathway of clotting factor is measured by:

a. Bleeding time
b. Prothrombin time
c. Activated partial thromboplastin time
d. Clotting time

Ans. b. Prothrombin time

(Ref: Guyton and Hall 13th edition, page 263)

Extrinsic pathway is measured by prothrombin time (PTT) whereas intrinsic pathway is measured by activated partial prothrombin time (APPT).

259. Earliest sign of vocal cord paralysis:

a. Rough voice quality
b. Hyperfunction
c. Diplophonia
d. Glottal insufficiency

Ans. a. Rough voice quality

(Ref: Guyton and Hall 13th edition, page 237)

- The most commonly reported symptom patients with either vocal fold paresis or paralysis make is having a rough voice quality.
- It is important to note that the symptoms of vocal fold paresis are not specific to the condition and tend to be common symptoms of other voice disorders as well.
- Vocal fold bowing, decreased vocal fold mobility, especially decreased mobility of the arytenoid cartilage, are often observed in vocal fold paresis.

260. 19 years old, Primi, 8 weeks gestation, presents with light bleeding otherwise normal. What is the next line of management?

a. Bed rest
b. D and C
c. Both
d. None

Ans. a. Bed rest *(Ref: DC Dutta's Textbook of Obstetrics 9th edition, page 452)*

- Bleeding can take place at around 6 to 8 weeks of gestation. The same can be true in pregnancy, with bleeding occurring around 8 weeks because the body is so used to bleeding each month.

- But unlike regular period blood, this bleeding is typically really light and limited to spotting or dark brown blood. So just continue bed rest is management of choice in this case.

261. Propofol TCI using Marsh model (in "Diprifusor") is affected by which of the following parameters?

a. Weight
b. Height
c. Age
d. Weight and height

Ans. d. Weight and height

(Ref: Morgan and Mikhail's Clinical Anesthesiology, 6th edition, page 122)

- Target-controlled infusion (TCI) systems can be programmed with any pharmacokinetic model, and allow either plasma- or effect-site targeting. With effect-site targeting the goal is to achieve a user-defined target effect-site concentration as rapidly as possible, by manipulating the plasma concentration around the target.
- Currently systems are pre-programmed with the Marsh and Schnider pharmacokinetic models for propofol.
- The former is an adapted version of the Gepts model, in which the rate constants are fixed, whereas compartment volumes and clearances are weight proportional.
- The Schneider model was developed during combined pharmacokinetic–pharmacodynamic modelling studies. It has fixed values for V1, V3, k13, and k31, adjusts V2, k12, and k21 for age, and adjusts k according to total weight, lean body mass (LBM), and height.

262. Diagnose the skin disease in the following picture:

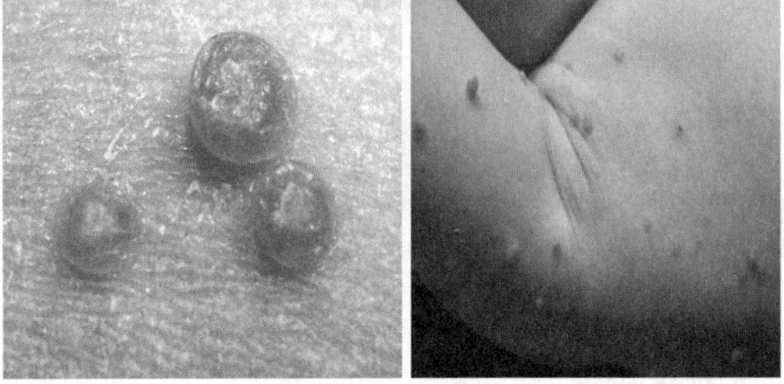

For color version see plate 1

a. Molluscum contagiosum
b. Basal-cell carcinoma
c. Acrochordons
d. Wart

Ans. a. Molluscum contagiosum

263. The following image is:

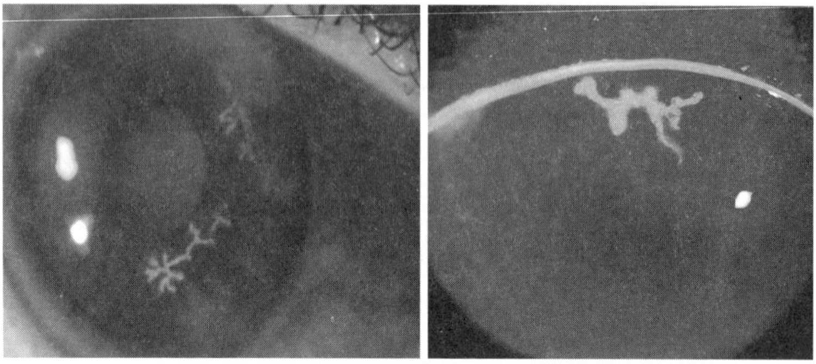

For color version see plate 1

a. Dendritic ulcer
b. Geographic ulcer
c. Disciform keratitis
d. Herpetic epithelial keratitis

Ans. d. Herpetic epithelial keratitis

264. X-ray showing:

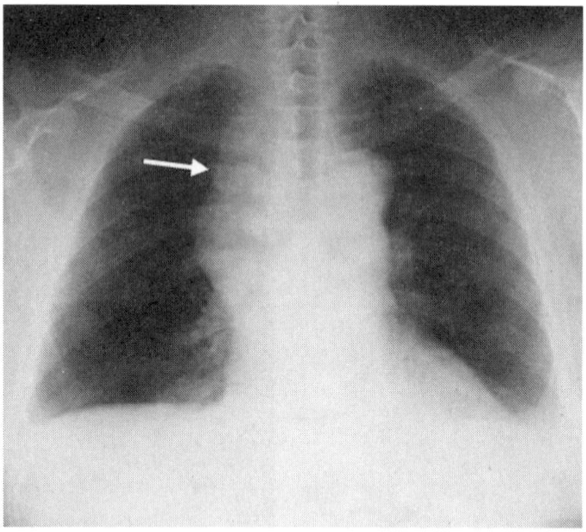

For high resolution see plate 2

a. Massive pleural effusion
b. Heart failure
c. Pulmonary embolism
d. Subpulmonic effusion

Ans. a. Massive pleural effusion

265. Which of the following is correct:

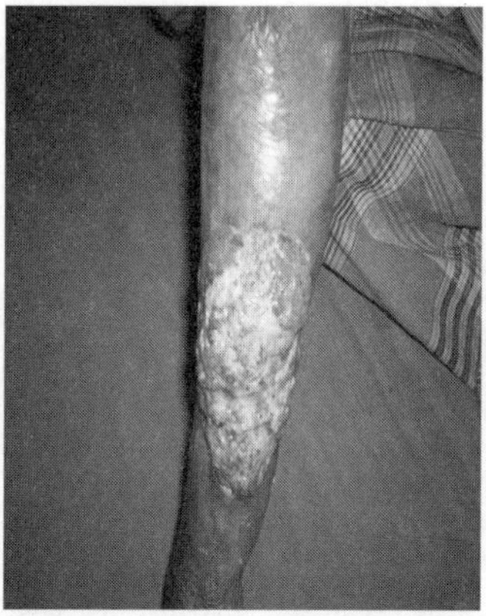

For color version see plate 2

a. Saree cancer
b. Marjolin ulcer
c. Venous ulcers
d. Rodent ulcer

Ans. b. Marjolin ulcer

266. Describe the following image:

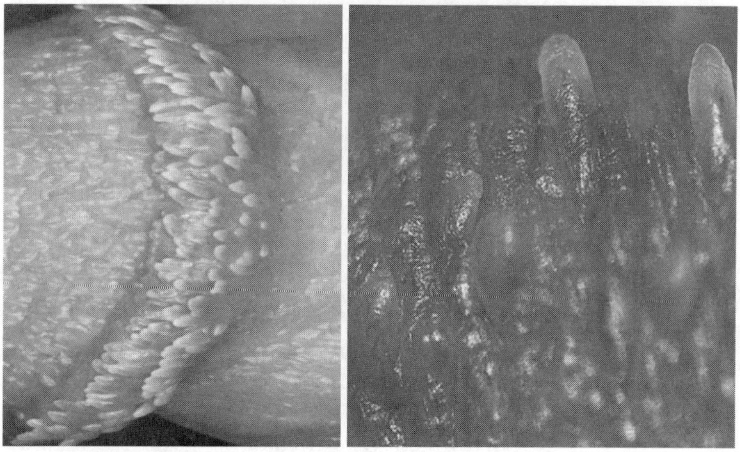

For color version see plate 3

a. Genital warts
b. Molluscum contagiosum
c. Lichen nitidus
d. Pearly penile papules

Ans. d. Pearly penile papules

267. Describe the following?

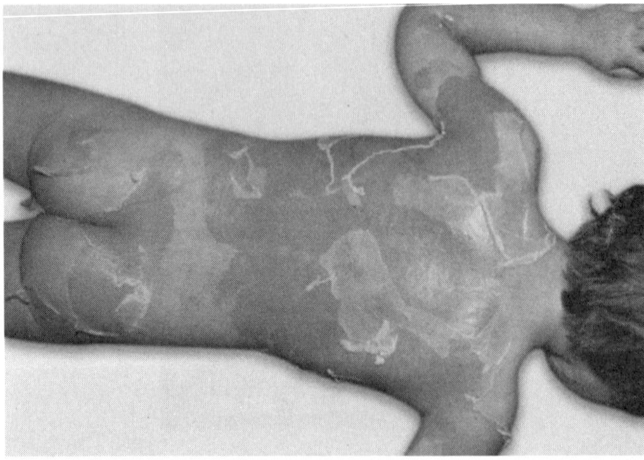

For color version see plate 3

a. Staphylococcal scalded skin syndrome
b. Acne conglobata
c. Erythrotelangiectatic rosacea
d. Granulomatous perioral dermatitis

Ans. a. Staphylococcal scalded skin syndrome

268. Please explain the picture:

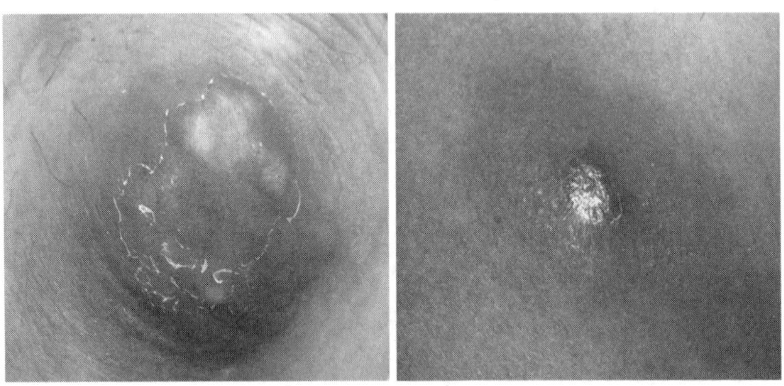

For color version see plate 4

a. Boils
b. Pilonidal cyst
c. Hidradenitis suppurativa
d. Cystic acne

Ans. a. Boils

269. X-ray picture shows:

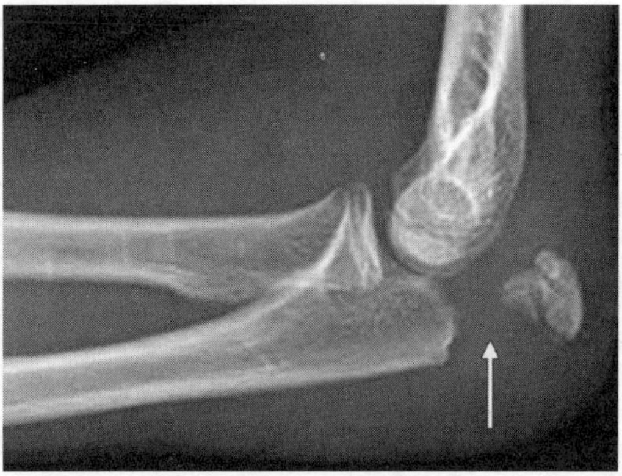

For high resolution see plate 4

a. Olecranon fracture
b. Supracondylar fracture
c. Physeal fractures
d. Monteggia fractures

Ans. a. Olecranon fracture

270. Which of the following is correct:

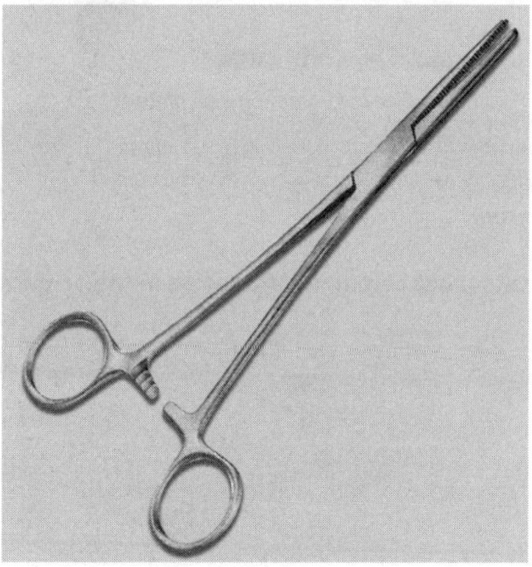

For color version see plate 5

a. Artery forcep
b. Mosquito forceps
c. Thumb forceps
d. Kelly forceps

Ans. a. Artery forcep

271. Describe the following image:

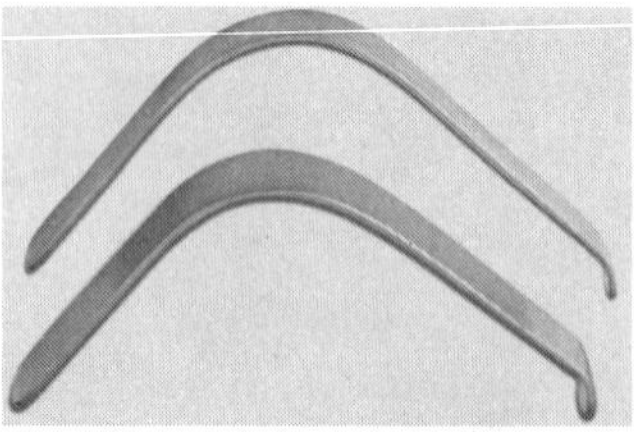

For color version see plate 5

a. Stick bomb grenade
b. Tongue depressor crafts
c. Lack Tongue Depressor
d. Stainless steel blade

Ans. c. Lack Tongue Depressor

272. Identify the slide:

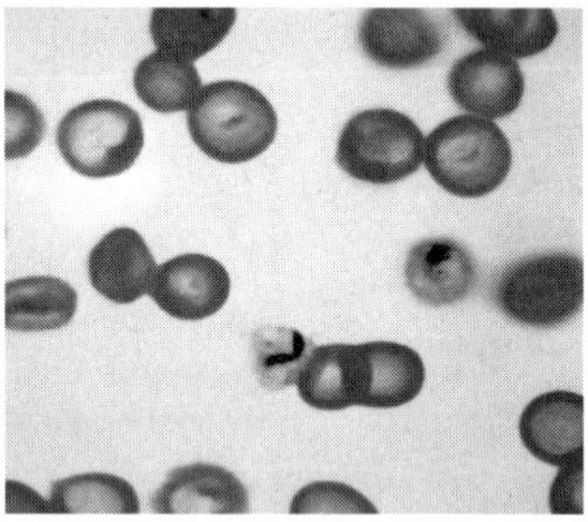

For color version see plate 6

a. *P. falciparum*
b. *P. vivax*
c. *P. malariae*
d. *P. ovale*

Ans. a. *P. falciparum*

273. Which bone is most commonly fractured in the arrow marked area?

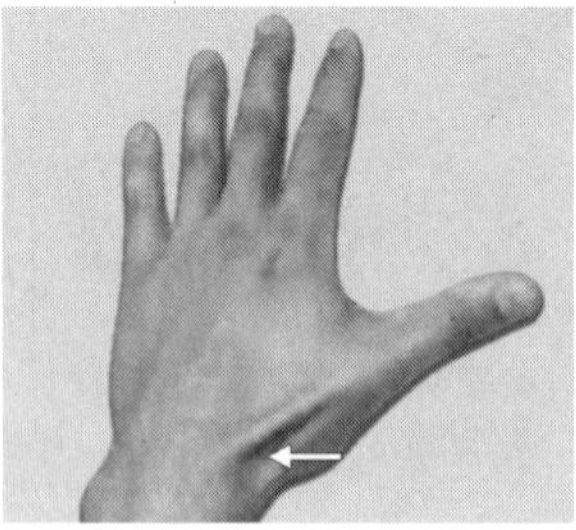

For color version see plate 6

a. Scaphoid
b. Extensor pollicis brevis
c. Extensor pollicis longus
d. Abductor pollicis longus

Ans. a. Scaphoid

274. Identify the muscle:

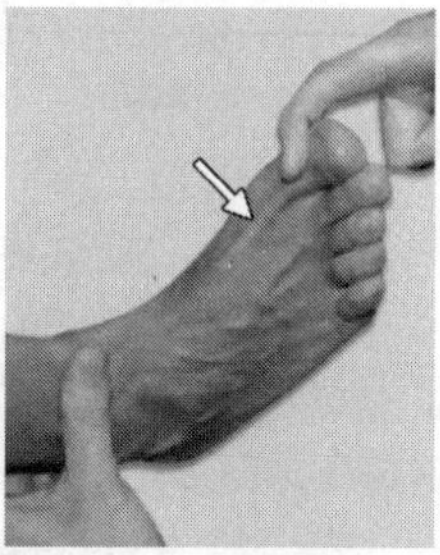

For color version see plate 7

a. Extensor digitorum brevis
b. Extensor hallucis brevis
c. Tibialis anterior
d. Extensor hallucis longus

Ans. d. Extensor hallucis longus

275. Identify the red marked muscle:

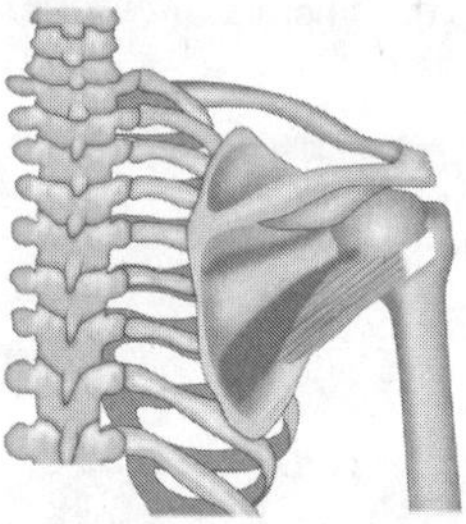

For color version see plate 7

a. Teres major
b. Teres minor
c. Infraspinatus
d. Supraspinatus

Ans. a. Teres major

276. Which is thls apparatus?

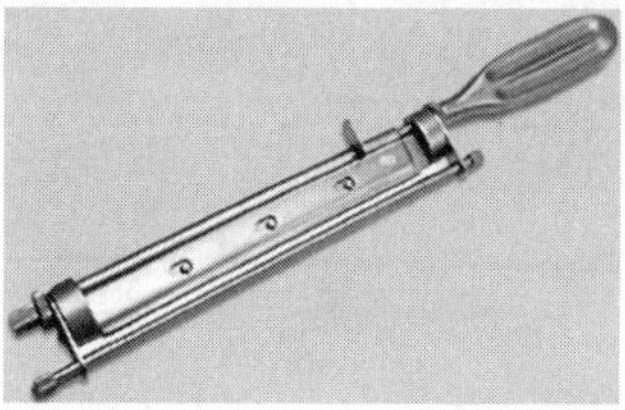

For color version see plate 8

a. Humphrey graft knife
b. Humby graft knife
c. Aesculap skin graft knife
d. Watson skin graft knife

Ans. d. Watson skin graft knife

277. X-ray shows:

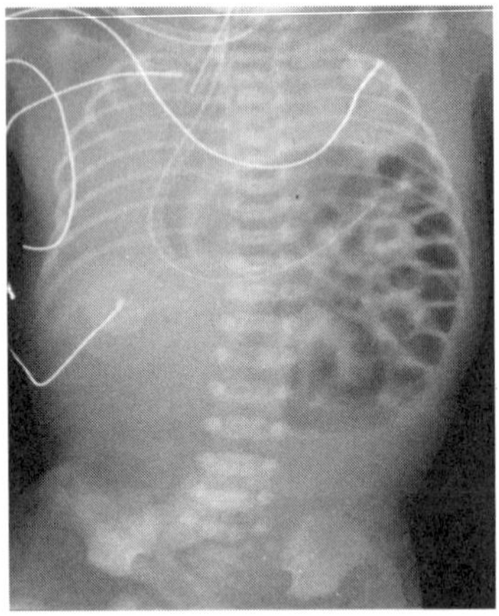

For high resolution see plate 8

a. Congenital diaphragmatic hernia
b. Pulmonary hypoplasia
c. Mediastinal shift
d. Phrenic nerve palsy

Ans. a. Congenital diaphragmatic hernia

278. X-ray picture shows:

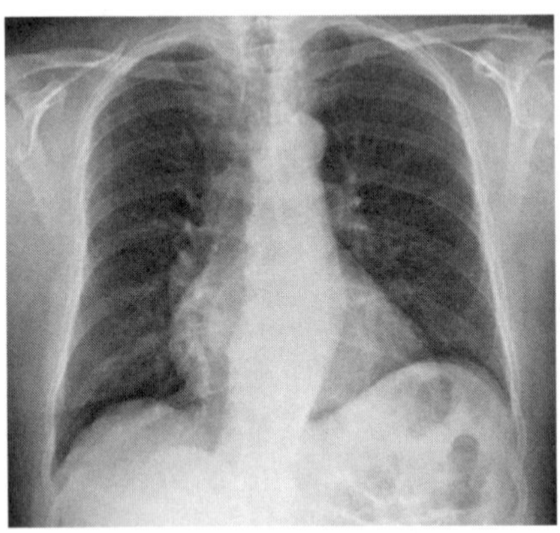

For high resolution see plate 9

a. Atrial septal defect
b. Prosthetic valve obstruction
c. Mitral regurgitation
d. Mitral stenosis

Ans. d. Mitral stenosis

279. Identify the picture:

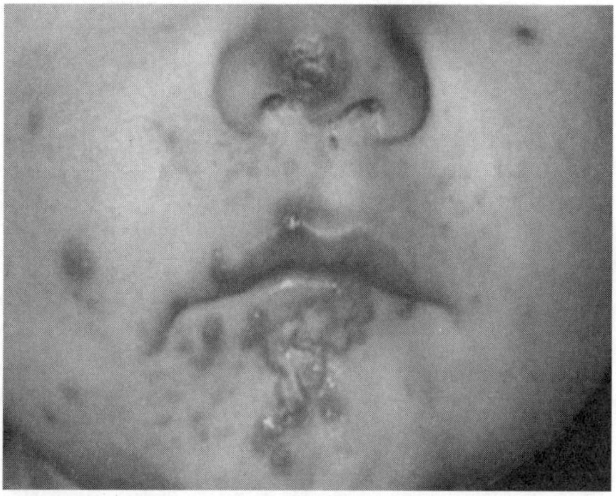

For color version see plate 9

a. Impetigo
b. Tinea
c. Varicella
d. Cutaneous candidiasis

Ans. a. Impetigo

280. Which of the following picture is correct?

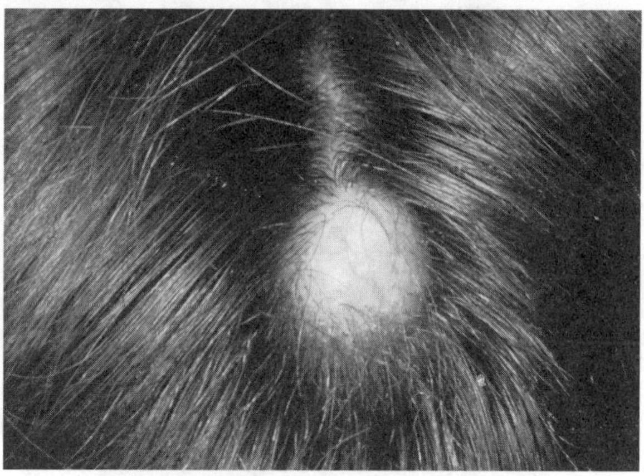

For color version see plate 10

a. Sebaceous cyst on scalp
b. Lipoma
c. Dermoid cyst on scalp
d. Epidermoid cysts on scalp

Ans. a. Sebaceous cyst on scalp

281. X-ray showing:

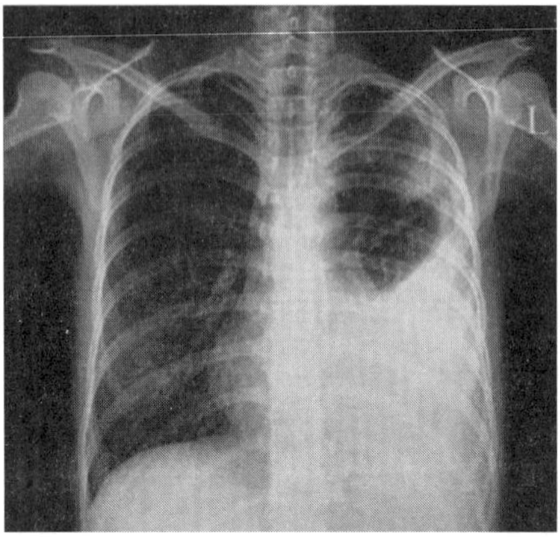

For high resolution see plate 10

a. Pleural effusion mild moderate severe
b. Malignant pleural effusions
c. Exudative pleural effusion
d. None of the above

Ans. b. Malignant pleural effusions

282. Which of the following is this?

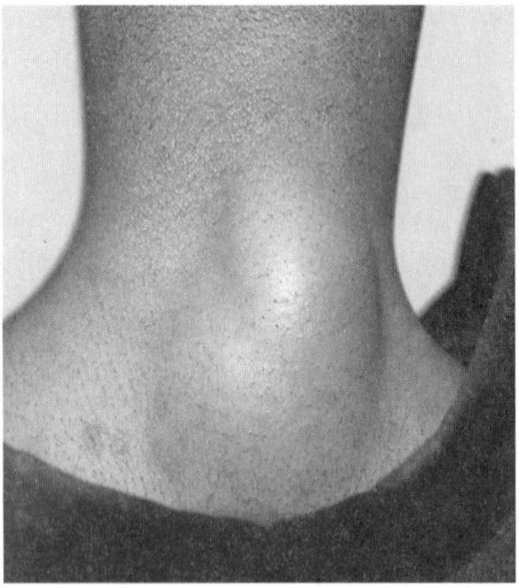

For color version see plate 11

a. Sebaceous cyst
b. An abscess
c. Lipoma
d. Atypical lipomatous tumor

Ans. c. Lipoma

283. The image given below leads to which muscle weakness?

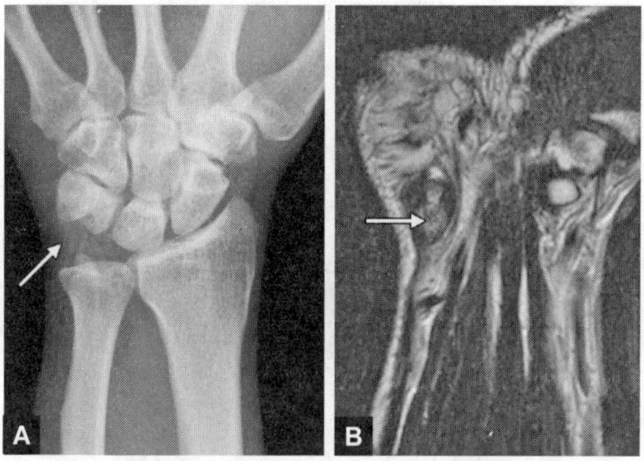

For high resolution see plate 11

a. Flexor carpi ulnaris
b. Extensor carpi ulnaris
c. Tendinous
d. None of the above

Ans. a. Flexor carpi ulnaris

284. True about the picture:

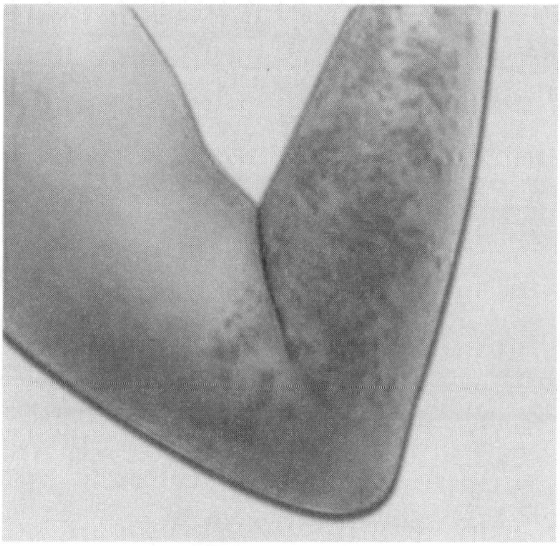

For color version see plate 12

a. Pityriasis alba
b. Tinea pedis
c. Psoriasis
d. Allergic contact dermatitis

Ans. c. Psoriasis

285. A child presents with bilious vomiting on day 2 of life and mother gives history of polyhydramnios. The radiological imaging is show. What is your probable diagnosis?

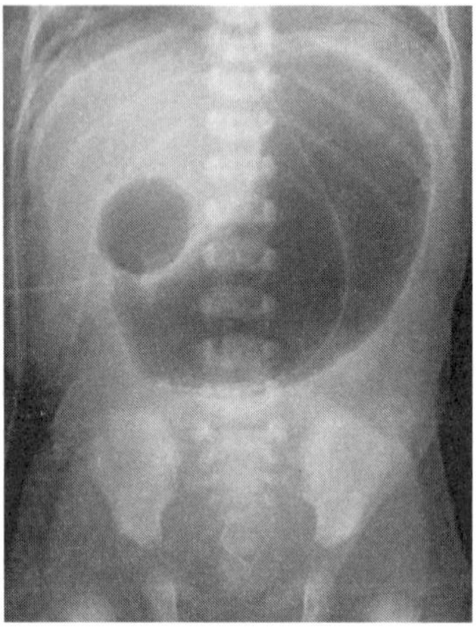

For high resolution see plate 12

a. Ileal atresia
b. Congenital mega colon
c. Duodenal atresia
d. Hypertrophic pyloric stenosis

Ans. c. Duodenal atresia